MW00474450

Brain
Weaver

Brain
Weaver

CREATING THE FABRIC FOR A HEALTHY MIND
THROUGH INTEGRATIVE MEDICINE

ANDREW NEWBERG, MD and
DANIEL A. MONTI, MD

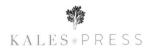

KALES·PRESS

in association with the

MARCUS INSTITUTE OF INTEGRATIVE HEALTH

Kenneth Kales, Editor
Barbara J. Greenberg, Associate Editor
Beverly Miller, Assistant Editor

Jacket design by Laura Klynstra
Interior design by Jennifer Houle

Copyright © 2021 by Andrew Newberg and Daniel A. Monti

Reproduced with permission: "The Sorcerer" by Breuil, Henri, 1877–1961. "Four hundred centuries of cave art. Translated by Mary E. Boyle. Realized by Fernand Windels." Rare Books. WCSU Archives.

Library of Congress Cataloging-in-Publication Data

Names: Newberg, Andrew B., 1966- author. | Monti, Daniel A., author.
Title: Brain weaver : creating the fabric for a healthy mind through integrative medicine / Andrew B. Newberg and Daniel A. Monti.
Description: First edition. | San Diego, California : Kales Press in association with the Marcus Institute of Integrative Health, [2021] | Includes index. | Summary: "Doctors Newberg and Monti's team at Jefferson University's Marcus Institute of Integrative Health is on the cutting edge of discoveries in brain functioning, and apply the most advanced concepts into real world strategies that expand options to ptimize complex neurophysiology based on the following approach: Optimal brain health = successfully weaving together a tapestry of our bio-psycho-social-spiritual dimensions. Being at the forefront of advances in neuroscience affords Doctors Newberg and Monti fresh perspective on mind-body functioning. Though adult cognitive development has previously been thought to be unyielding and static, Brain Weaver offers new hope and empowerment for adults to remain mentally vibrant for a lifetime by incorporating the principles of Integrative Medicine"—Provided by publisher.
Identifiers: LCCN 2020057948 (print) | LCCN 2020057949 (ebook) | ISBN 9781733395816 (cloth) | ISBN 9781733395823 (ebook)
Subjects: LCSH: Neuropsychiatry--Popular works. | Brain--Care and hygiene. | Mind and body. | Integrative medicine.
Classification: LCC RC343 .N485 2021 (print) | LCC RC343 (ebook) | DDC 616.8—dc23
LC record available at https://lccn.loc.gov/2020057948
LC ebook record available at https://lccn.loc.gov/2020057949

Printed in the United States of America

First Edition

ISBN-13: 978-1-7333958-1-6 print edition
ISBN-13: 978-1-7333958-2-3 ebook edition

kalespress.com
San Diego, California

To the tremendous colleagues, partners, and patients
who helped us create a cutting-edge platform for brain-body healing

The Brain is wider than the Sky

—Emily Dickinson

CONTENTS

PART TWO: HEALING SYSTEMS

PART THREE: DEALING WITH BRAIN PROBLEMS

FOREWORD

The pivotal moments in my life have been guided by a profound sense of knowing when the current way of doing something could be rethought and retooled. This is what led to my conceptualization of the Home Depot, and it is why my nonprofit foundation, the Marcus Institute of Integrative Health, has invested considerable resources in the field of integrative medicine. In both cases, the system was not fully meeting the needs of its customers. The latter is the basis of this book, and the authors, Dr. Andrew Newberg and Dr. Daniel Monti, have become a personal part of my life and wellness journey. This is particularly the case for the author of the book's Introduction, Dr. George Zabrecky, who has been the most influential person in terms of how I think about medicine and health care outside the box of the Western system. Dr. Zabrecky is a maverick thinker, as are the two lead authors, which is why the innovative programs at the Marcus Institute of Integrative Health at Thomas Jefferson University are like nothing else in the world.

Brain Weaver offers a fresh perspective on achieving optimal brain health by providing the science behind the Marcus Institute's comprehensive approaches in a reader-friendly format. It teaches that the parts can never be greater than the whole and that we must think about the entire human system when considering the health and functioning of the brain. The authors have accomplished this by elegantly weaving all of the components that science has revealed into one cohesive plan that can benefit us all. I believe this book will make a big difference in human lives, and I am recommending it to everyone in my close circle. As the US population ages, it is essential for all of us to have the best cutting-edge information to think our best, feel our best, and function at our best. The revolutionary research and clinical practices this book explores have been developed from the tremendous partnership between Thomas Jefferson University and the Marcus Foundation.

The book is written to engage you as the creator of your best brain and to think beyond the traditional medical standards to include all of the approaches that might give you the edge needed to outperform the you of fifteen years ago.

This book also has the potential to change the overall culture of medicine by showing doctors and patients alike the best way to optimize brain health. The authors explain the high-level research they've conducted using the most technologically advanced equipment available to assess the brain's reactivity to lifestyle interventions, targeted nutrient therapies, complementary approaches, and integrated care plans. Newberg, Monti, and Zabrecky are at the cutting edge of this work: they established the first ever Department of Integrative Medicine and Nutritional Sciences at a traditional medical school, a truly paradigm-shifting event. As leaders in the field and compassionate clinicians, they work to educate the next generation of doctors and to make sure that patients are empowered to pursue the best health care possible, working in tandem with their physicians.

These authors have a great ability to study the brain and translate their knowledge into a tangible prescription for brain health. They of course follow modern science, yet they are not afraid to explore options beyond traditional medicine in order to help as many people as possible. They also understand the importance of looking at evidence-based medicine and bringing that information to every patient. That is the basis of *Brain Weaver*. It is with books like this that we hope the future of medicine will advance to include the best of current practices, lifestyle medicine, and novel integrative therapies so that we all can maintain and even improve our body and brain's health for as long as possible.

Bernie Marcus
Cofounder of The Home Depot

INTRODUCTION

Plato recognized two kinds of mental disease: madness and ignorance. He believed that much of the vice is due to the ill disposition of the body and is involuntary: "For no man is voluntarily bad; but the bad became bad by reason of ill disposition of the body and bad education, things which are hateful to every man and happen to him against his will."

Brain Weaver educates readers in comprehending the many causes of "ill disposition" and how supportive integrative medicine is fundamental, even critical in many cases, to the best brain health achievable. Integrative medicine refers to an approach that incorporates conventional medicine with evidence-based complementary and alternative methods including diet and nutrition, mind-body practices, botanical products, and other related therapies.

Dr. Newberg and Dr. Monti have done a tremendous job encapsulating the best of integrative medicine in the context of brain health. I know that these physicians, close, personal colleagues of mine, are passionate about every individual they encounter, and they always strive to give their patients the best possible guidance to weave their best brains possible. One of the fundamental aspects of their approach is to recognize that each of us is a multidimensional person who needs every aspect of ourselves to be taken into consideration. For some people, their biology is fine, but they lack a strong social support network. Others have great friends and family but a terrible diet. It is important that each of us learns to work with our strengths and shortcomings, and how to do that is exactly what you will find in *Brain Weaver*.

This book works to establish a new paradigm of brain health that starts with the basics—your genetics and your environment, along with your diet and nutrition. It then expands greatly to help you understand how these many factors affect the brain, how to manage them properly, and what to do when the brain is not working well. With a great deal of information and step-by-step recommendations, Newberg and Monti show you the best of what modern medicine, including integrative medicine, has to offer.

This revolution in brain health is just beginning. It is starting at places like the Department of Integrative Medicine and Nutritional Sciences at Thomas Jefferson University, home of the Marcus Institute of Integrative Health. But it is expanding rapidly around the world. Integrative medicine and integrative brain health are continuing to make their mark on the scientific community. With more and more research and clinical care, we are understanding how integrative medicine will become, simply, "medicine," and how integrative brain health will become, simply, "brain health." What is important is for each of us to be empowered to create our own personal, dynamic, and thriving program to weave our optimal brain.

Andrew Newberg and Daniel Monti are among the elite physician-researchers in the world, and the work they do has tremendous credibility. Their expertise is highly individualized and at the same time overlaps in just the ways needed to propel the field forward. Together, they provide a diversity and uniqueness of academic and clinical medicine that pave the way for an understanding of brain health that is innovative and results oriented.

Newberg completed medical school at the University of Pennsylvania and is board certified in both internal medicine and nuclear medicine. He has pursued a large number of neuroimaging research projects that have included the study of aging and dementia, epilepsy, and other neurological and psychiatric disorders. He has intensively studied the more general mind-body relationship in both the clinical and research aspects of his career, including understanding the physiological correlates of acupuncture therapy, meditation, and other types of integrative therapies. He has published over 250 peer-reviewed articles and chapters on brain function, brain imaging, and the study of neurological and psychiatric conditions. He was listed as one of the 30 Most Influential Neuroscientists Alive Today by the Online Psychology Degree Guide.

Monti completed a research scholars program after medical school, and his training and work have focused on psychiatry, mind-body health, and the role of natural molecules on neurocognitive and immune outcomes. He is the founding chair of the Department of Integrative Medicine and Nutritional Sciences at Jefferson. He has authored dozens of scholarly articles, medical textbooks, and popular press writings. He has performed landmark studies on various nutrient molecules such as the use of N-acetylcysteine, a powerful antioxidant, in patients with multiple sclerosis, Parkinson's disease, and traumatic brain injuries and is currently completing a study on the role of vitamin C in COVID-19 outcomes. He has been at the forefront of studying mind-body interventions, including the Neuro Emotional Technique and mindfulness-based practices.

GEORGE ZABRECKY, DC, MD
ACADEMIC DIRECTOR, MARCUS INSTITUTE OF
INTEGRATIVE HEALTH–JEFFERSON HEALTH

PART ONE

The Basics

Chapter 1

A NEW PARADIGM FOR HEALING

The soul heals and science cures.

—MYRNA BRIND, 2003

Let's start with a simple question: How would you define your optimal brain health?

As experts on cognitive function, we know you have probably thought about this and that, consciously or not, you might even have an idea of what your ideal brain health would be like. The science we are about to present, along with evidence-based, practical strategies for maximizing your brain health potential, are best understood when considered within the context of your individual goals and aspirations. Ask yourself what those are for you. Everyone is different. For a twenty-year-old college student, it might be performing well on final exams. For a thirty-year-old parent of two kids, it might be keeping sane just long enough at the end of the day to get them to sleep and still having enough in reserve to check a favorite social media site or read a book. For a fifty-year-old businessperson, it might be controlling stress and staying focused amid the intense financial vagaries of the business world. For a sixty-two-year-old, it might be restoring some of the cognitive sharpness that has gotten sluggish. And for an eighty-year-old, it might be protecting against dementia and having a fantastic quality of life that includes playing with grandchildren or great-grandchildren.

As you begin to think about your answer to this critical question, we want to put the notion of optimal brain health in the appropriate perspective—one that is protective, proactive, and preserving. We will introduce you to an integrative approach that draws on a diverse set of data implemented in a practical way that makes sense.

Our approach contrasts with the medical model that is solely disease focused, disjointed, incohesive, and reactive. In that model, you see a medical doctor mostly for symptoms of physical illnesses, a psychotherapist for your mental and emotional struggles, and a spiritual adviser for matters of the soul such as your religious or sacred values, purpose, or meaning in life. In addition, you might seek the advice of the local health food store clerk for your diet and supplements and scour the Internet to fill the ever-growing gap spanning what doesn't get addressed by all of the above.

We are proposing a fresh perspective that we have constructed and tested from our years of integrative medicine practice and research. Our new paradigm recognizes that your psychological, social, and spiritual dimensions are as important as, if not more important than, the biological ones in the healing process of your brain and body. The brain is a component of the body, and every cell that comprises who you are is elegantly connected in a network more sophisticated than that of any computer. This new paradigm recognizes that the architecture of you has a vast number of points of entry for healing—everything from the activities you choose to the foods you eat. Our therapeutic approach goes far beyond a pill we could prescribe and instead is geared to have an impact on the way you will think, function, feel, and thrive for many years to come.

We need this new approach to brain health of integrating the best of modern science and modern medicine and including the other facets of life that affect the complex networks of our unique humanity. This approach does not exclusively rely on medications, or exclusively focus on the power of the mind, or even rely just on the values to be found in ancient wisdom. Instead, our new paradigm embraces a fully integrative model that uses all of these sources, blending them with the latest findings in neuroscience and distilling them into a plan that can be life changing. We have pioneered this model at the Marcus Institute of Integrative

Health at Thomas Jefferson University, where we have developed cutting-edge, groundbreaking programs and protocols in the world.

This new journey requires us to change our overall definition of optimal brain health. In fact, throughout this book, we offer three perspectives on what optimal brain health is:

#1. Optimal Brain Health =
Biological + Psychological + Social + Spiritual Health

Most brain health approaches focus on only one or two of these key factors. but our research has shown the importance of all of them and also how each of them plays off the others. Hence, we need an integrative approach that recognizes the importance of each of these components of optimal brain health and engages them actively. There is strong science now to support our proposed, which is critical to achieving the best results.

Modern medicine primarily focuses on the biological component, and even then, it does so in a way that emphasizes drugs to address symptoms of disease, with little attention to establishing resilience and functional wellness. For many people, here's the dilemma: modern medicine isn't completely wrong. In fact, in the appropriate situation, it can be the only thing that can save your life. If you have an acute injury like a broken bone or need stitches, the best place for you is in the hands of competent physicians. However, establishing and enhancing wellness, preventing disease, integrating all the lifestyle variables that contribute to how you think, function, and feel, are not what conventional modern medicine shines at. We understand that when it comes to the complexities of brain health, the medical model on its own is too limited. Yet approaches outside the medical model aren't completely right either, especially when they are considered in isolation of good medical care. What we do throughout this book is show you how to integrate modern medical science with innovative healing arts that have been confirmed by the most recent scientific evidence. We have done the research, and our team has published widely in these domains. Our approach is designed to empower you to improve your health status and achieve optimal brain health now and throughout your entire life.

So let's go back to that question: What do you perceive to be your optimal brain health? In fact, write it down so you know as clearly as possible what your answer is. Start by taking out a piece of paper, making sure there is room for at least about ten lines of writing. Put the paper on the table in front of you and sit down with a pen or pencil—or open up the notes app on your smartphone or a Word document on your computer. Now take a few deep breaths and clear your mind of any thoughts you have. Then ask yourself, *What do I think represents my optimal brain health?* Write down whatever comes into your mind—a sentence or a word. Maybe it is something like "sharpness" or "mental clarity." Maybe it is, "I want to be more positive and less depressed." If you write something down that is negative like, "I don't want Alzheimer's!" rewrite it into a positive statement such as, "I want to avoid Alzheimer's as much as I can." There is a reason to state things positively, but we will get to that a little later on. For now, focus on creating a positive, proactive picture of your aspirational brain health.

Next, let's take a snapshot of your current brain-body health status. Since the two are inextricably connected, the health of one is directly connected to the health of the other. Take an inventory of what you consider to be strengths and weaknesses in your own brain-body architecture. For example, do you have any chronic conditions or diseases? If so, how are you managing those conditions? Do you take medications for your brain or for other medical conditions? Are there ways that you excel physically or mentally? What is your current stress level, and how stressful is your life in general? Do you have a terrific memory for names? Do you eat a healthy diet? Do you exercise regularly? Is your weight where you want it to be? You do not have to write all of these things down, but it is important to keep in mind who you are and what comprises your unique biology. Our program meets you where you are. It is important to note where that is so we can objectively chart the results as you take the reins of your brain health destiny. Everything we will examine in this book must be considered in the context of your own life—your own personal strengths and challenges.

STRATEGY: ENHANCE STRENGTHS; TRANSFORM VULNERABILITIES

A key strategy to our path to optimal brain health is to teach you how to maximize your strengths and find ways of bolstering perceived and real weaknesses and vulnerabilities, and correcting them when possible. It is helpful now to take a take a deeper dive into how you perceive your own personal strengths and weaknesses with regard to brain health. The brain has an incredible array of abilities, so let's spend some time reflecting on all of the possible ways you use your brain so you can see where you shine and where you may need some extra attention may be needed.

We start with a brief introduction to cognitive processes that we build on in later chapters. This will help us assess your personal baseline. We start with self-reflection, an important exercise to do regularly. Reflect for a moment on the way your own memory system is constructed and whether you can identify strengths in how your memory works and for what types of things. Do you remember things in your own life, like what happened at events or what you wore to an important first date? Do you have a knack for numbers or names? Were you a good student because you had raw memory or because you could solve problems creatively? Perhaps you know your IQ or have taken an IQ test online. These all give you some sense as to what you are starting with. You might have answered affirmatively to one, none, or all of these. The important thing is that you reflect on these dimensions of memory. But one thing is for sure: if you are reading this book, you have proficiencies. All too often, we focus on deficits or vulnerabilities, but those are only a small part of who we are. The totality of you has a great deal of vibrant untapped potential. Our goal is to determine what has emerged and then help you unlock the rest. Vulnerabilities may always be there, but the good news is that we can minimize them by bolstering strengths and creating resilience around areas that feel less solid. Just taking inventory as we are suggesting can help us arrive at strategies.

For example, I (Andy) was never good at names, and it felt like a real impediment all through college and medical school. By applying our principle of self-reflection, I am also aware that I am very good at remembering associations. This self-reflection, along with other strategies we will be discussing, has helped me to improve this deficit significantly while strengthening the rest of my brain health. By leveraging my self-assessed strengths, I began to use ways of linking a person's name with other characteristics of the person that are easier for me to remember, such as what that person does for a living or how the name of that person's company correlates with his or her name: for example, Jeffrey is from Jefferson.

Our goal is to help you think through your strengths and challenges as part of the overall strategy of performing better and improving your quality of life. Beyond this simple cognitive task, I was aware of developing a kind of anxiety around recalling peoples' names. I realized I had to address getting overly discouraged when I had trouble with this. Recognizing these issues, I learned some of the advanced mind-body techniques we discuss in *Brain Weaver*. Another important insight from my self-reflection on what I was calling a memory problem was that the whole issue became exponentially worse when I was in low blood sugar mode. I addressed this with some of the same dietary strategies we discuss in upcoming chapters. The multipronged, integrative approach in this simple example has led me to being much better at navigating names in social situations, and as a result improved my overall quality of life. In fact, many people around me now tell me that I am quite good at remembering names.

A LITTLE BIT MORE ON HOW MEMORY WORKS

Much of memory starts with the hippocampus, a structure in the brain. The hippocampus, which is Greek for "sea horse" as a description of its shape, is part of the brain's limbic system, our emotional center, and is involved in helping us to remember information. It's also one of the first brain areas to go in disorders such as Alzheimer's disease. What is interesting is that chronic states of stress can damage the hippocampus and that the novel stress reduction techniques we discuss in upcoming chapters can improve hippocampus functioning. There also is exciting emerging research suggesting that dietary factors and exercise can have a direct impact on the hippocampus, which we also discuss in detail.

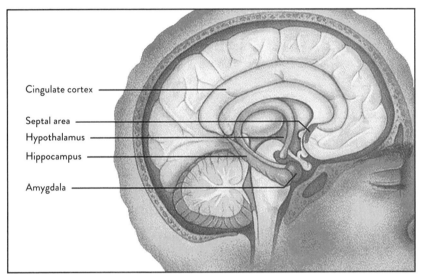

Structure of the limbic system.
ILLUSTRATION COURTESY OF THE MARCUS INSTITUTE OF INTEGRATIVE HEALTH

Another dimension of brain function, and hence brain health, is language. This becomes more obvious in situations where the language centers of the brain are damaged by something like a stroke or brain injury or in a disease process like Alzheimer's. More subtle changes can occur during aging, which underscores why reflecting on your own baseline is important. Like other dimensions of brain function, our language capabilities can be strengthened or impeded by factors that are in our control.

Language is not only about having a good vocabulary, but knowing when to use the right words, particularly in complicated or difficult situations. The language parts of the brain are divided into receptive and expressive areas, and they do exactly what their names suggest. The receptive areas, located along the side of the brain in what is called the temporal lobe, receive words and help us understand them when we hear or see them. The expressive areas, located near the front of the brain in what is called Broca's area, help us produce speech in order to say what we are thinking. These areas are connected so we can hear what someone is saying, understand it, develop a response, and reply to the person. The language areas are generally on the left side of the brain but can be distributed across both sides, particularly in people who are left-handed. Other regions of the brain help with the nonverbal parts of language such as facial expression and body language. Protecting all of these areas is important for maintaining your ability to interact with other people and communicate well.

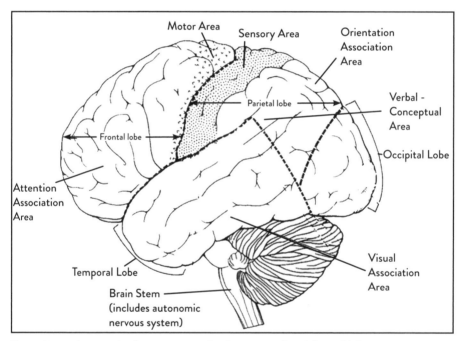

Receptive and expressive language areas in the temporal and frontal lobes.
ILLUSTRATION COURTESY OF THE MARCUS INSTITUTE OF INTEGRATIVE HEALTH

The executive functions, which make us uniquely human, arise mostly from the frontal lobes and are involved in helping you maintain all of the basic aspects of daily life, such as setting and following your schedule, planning your lunch, keeping your finances in order, and going on a vacation. Some people are particularly well organized in life and maintain a highly structured plan through-out their job, relationships, and activities. Others don't have a frontal lobe that keeps things as structured, and sometimes they can appear less organized or even a bit flaky and scattered. Being too highly organized can lead to obsessive-compulsive behaviors, and not being organized enough can make leading a nor-mal life difficult. As with most other things in life, a proper balance is always the best, and maintaining that balance is an important part of optimal brain health.

YOUR EMOTIONAL BRAIN

Emotions are a function of the brain, that is, they are neurological. At one time, their physical components were much more elusive and intangible, which is one of the reasons mind and body were seen as being separate not so long ago. Emotional dysregulation now can be seen when the brain is damaged, and some of the more subtle changes in emotional well-being can be identified as a reflec-tion of imbalances in nutritional biochemistry, illness, stress overload, excessive inflammation, and more. This aspect of brain function and health is crucial to evaluate because your emotional state can have a direct impact on how well you remember, process information, and perform cognitively. Beyond that, long-term unchecked stress levels can have measurable effects on the biology of the brain, including the amount of healthy brain tissue available in key regions of cognitive functioning. Research we have done at the Marcus Institute of Integrative Health has transformed the way we consider this relationship between emotional factors and cognition. Hence, emotional state is an important measure of how your brain is doing. If you are too stressed, too irritable, or too depressed, your brain is not in balance, and that usually has far-reaching effects, including on cognition. Currently, it appears that up to 20 percent of Americans will have some mental health issues in their life. The question is how best to protect yourself and help manage any emotional struggles you might have.

In addition, it is important to understand your general emotional set point, emotional intelligence, and whether your typical emotional responses in given situations act as assets or liabilities. For example, some great athletes are able to use their emotions to their advantage, particularly in stressful situations. One of the greatest women tennis players, Martina Navratilova, used to say, "Pressure is a privilege," meaning that if she felt emotional pressure, she was doing something good. And then she built off that emotional pressure to push herself to play even better. Other players react differently to pressure and use mental techniques to distance themselves from it. How you respond to stressors is part of your unique biology and psychology, which is why it is important for your path forward that you do an honest assessment. This is a time to take some stock of how you handle pressure and stressors in life. Do you excel in these situations? Or does your stomach get all tangled up in knots?

In addition, emotions themselves have a biology and biochemistry that can have an impact on the rest of your physiology. Emotions, a hard-wired aspect of the brain, serve an important role in survival. For example, happiness and love brings us together, fear helps us avoid harm, grief gives us a sense of loss that can be important for a community to work, and so on. In general, we all seek a balance between positive and negative emotions that enable us to navigate successfully through life. The problem in today's hurried society is that it often gets us overly stuck in so-called negative emotional states and doesn't allow us the time to balance them with the good physiological effects of so-called positive emotions.

Have you thought about what makes you happy or depressed? The positive emotions of joy, enjoyment, pride, interest, and excitement contribute to the emotional state we call happiness. This state has a biology to it that is important for health, including brain health. Since life will always have challenges associated with the negative emotions that detract, such as fear, anger, grief, worry, and shame, it is important to find the things in life that foster the positive ones. In upcoming chapters, we provide you with techniques to reset your brain to a positive emotional state. Some people find happiness by connecting with nature, for example, walking in the woods or, as the old John Denver song said, having sunshine on your shoulders can make you happy. Some find that creative expression in, say, painting or playing an instrument does the trick. Others get to happiness through high-thrill sports like downhill skiing. Do you get happy from a day lolling on the beach, or do you need to engage in spine-tingling activities like mountain climbing or skydiving to fulfill your emotional needs? Carving out time for the things that make you happy is an important consideration for brain health. But that is not always enough, so you need other tools (we will discuss them).

What causes your mood to get low? Here, we are talking about the normal ups and downs of life versus mania and clinical depression. Reflecting on the life situations that drag you down is important for context and also for applying techniques to improve your mind-body well-being. In what situations do you find you are making judgmental self-statements? Maybe your Achilles' heel is being in situations you can't control. Or does too much social isolation give you a depressed spirit? We address all of these, but the following simple test will help you get started on self-reflection.

This test will help you assess which of your brain processes are bolstering or hindering you. Answer the questions on a scale of 1 (Disagree) to 10 (Agree)— and be as honest with yourself as possible.

I find happiness in many aspects of life.

DISAGREE									AGREE
1	2	3	4	5	6	7	8	9	10

Quiet times with nature make me happy.

DISAGREE									AGREE
1	2	3	4	5	6	7	8	9	10

Intense activities such as rock climbing or skiing make me happy.

DISAGREE									AGREE
1	2	3	4	5	6	7	8	9	10

Spending time with friends and loved ones makes me happy.

DISAGREE									AGREE
1	2	3	4	5	6	7	8	9	10

I have a low mood much of the time.

DISAGREE									AGREE
1	2	3	4	5	6	7	8	9	10

My stress feels out of control.

DISAGREE									AGREE
1	2	3	4	5	6	7	8	9	10

I feel that I have control in my work life.

DISAGREE									AGREE
1	2	3	4	5	6	7	8	9	10

I feel that I have control in my personal life.

DISAGREE									AGREE
1	2	3	4	5	6	7	8	9	10

I have a good memory for names.

DISAGREE									AGREE
1	2	3	4	5	6	7	8	9	10

I have a good memory for numbers.

DISAGREE									AGREE
1	2	3	4	5	6	7	8	9	10

I have a large vocabulary.

DISAGREE									AGREE
1	2	3	4	5	6	7	8	9	10

Now carefully reflect on your answer to each of these questions and think about how they have an impact on your overall life. The numbers themselves reflect how strongly you feel about each of these brain processes. The ones that are contributing to a satisfying life are the current strengths in your life. The ones that detract from your happiness are the current weaknesses that are getting in the way. Don't worry or judge yourself if you have more weaknesses than strengths right now. Just try to write down two concise sentences—one that identifies your strengths and the other that states your goals for optimal brain health:

My brain strengths include _____

My brain health goals include _____

Throughout this book, we will help you harness your brain's abilities to improve. That is one of the great things about the brain: it can make itself better. And this leads us to the second perspective on defining optimal brain health.

#2. Optimal Brain Health = Neuroplasticity + the Dynamic Brain

---

THE WHOLE OF THE BRAIN IS
GREATER THAN THE SUM OF ITS PARTS

By cohesively using all of the components and functions of the brain, the neuronal connections that exist can adapt, change, and strengthen themselves. This process, referred to as *neuroplasticity*, means that the brain can keep changing. Although the brain changes most when you are young, you *can* teach an old dog new tricks. If you start to learn to play an instrument or you start studying history even when you are eighty years old, your brain can learn these new things. And learning is one of the best ways to make your brain better.

Two well-known sayings help explain how neuroplasticity works. "Neurons that fire together, wire together" means that the more you use a given set of neurons to do something—play an instrument, solve puzzles, or read about history, for example—the more the neurons that support those processes become connected and the stronger those connections become. That also goes for innovative problem solving such as learning new stress reduction skills. On the flip side, if you get lulled into bad habits or negative ideas, the neurology of those negative processes gets strengthened, leading to poorer brain function. In many ways, you are what you think. There are tremendous benefits to strengthening neuronal connections that will be to your advantage.

The second saying, "Use it or lose it," is fundamental to brain health because the less you use your brain and the less you use certain parts of it, the weaker those connections become. If you have learned to play the piano but don't go back to it for a year, you will slowly lose your ability to play. And if you don't challenge your memory and problem-solving abilities, you will lose them too. Technology can be a double-edged sword in this regard since our smartphones sometimes make us less smart. If you always use your GPS or if you speed-dial phone numbers without remembering them, you will lose the ability to find your way or remember your friend's phone number.

But if you consciously try to change how your brain works—for example, by learning some of the effective strategies we will teach you to create a positive effect in your life—the neuronal connections that support the more negative approaches will lessen with time, and new connection pathways will form and strengthen. We emphasize throughout this book how to take advantage of the ways in which you can get your brain to work better by fostering new, health-promoting neurological pathways.

THE NEW PARADIGM

We are at the forefront of up-to-the-minute advances in neuroscience, and this makes it possible for us to give you a fresh perspective on mind-body functioning. We now understand that the adult brain, previously thought to be unyielding and static, can be vibrant, ever-changing, and transforming. Our message is one of hope and excitement about the possibilities for your brain health, and also one of empowerment to incorporate tools that can transform the way you function and thrive.

Today's new science is replacing the long-standing paradigm in medicine that focuses almost exclusively on disjointed mechanisms of brain function with limited options for restoring or optimizing health. We are proposing an entirely different model: one that fully embraces all aspects of brain health and leads to optimal brain functioning, whether you have specific challenges or concerns or are just trying to build and maintain excellent brain capacity.

Our balanced perspective appreciates the incredible advances by modern medicine in the treatment of acute injury, surgical repairs, and many infectious diseases. However, the integrative approach that includes diet and nutrition, mind-body practices, and various nonmedical interventions is essential for good brain health. In fact, often the shortcoming in optimizing brain health and functioning is that it is sought out only after the frontline options of medication and surgery have either been exhausted or deemed inappropriate for the situation. For example, when dealing with challenges like cognitive decline, mood disorders, fatigue, and insomnia, the medicines and treatments prescribed typically have little or no effect and might even be harmful to your overall health. This is an issue when treating many chronic health conditions as well as when determining preventive care, and is especially the case when focusing on achieving optimal brain health.

The good news is that our fresh perspective on achieving optimal brain health is supported by extensive research, some of which we have conducted ourselves over the past ten years. Throughout this book, we invite you to expand your thinking as we help you envision the best possible approach to optimal brain health.

The new integrative medicine model that many of our colleagues have helped to develop has these important key elements:

1. *Biological*: How do you feed your brain? Are you getting the right nutrients? Starting with the right diet is essential for optimal brain health. We will describe the best diet to follow, focusing on foods that support brain health, reduce inflammation, and strengthen the brain-gut relationship.

We also discuss how to balance medications that might be necessary for you with natural alternatives, vitamins, and supplements that can help you achieve optimal brain health.

2. *Emotional/psychological*: How stressed is your brain? Do you have effective ways to lessen the burden life puts on your nervous system? We will describe the best approaches to adopt for enhancing psychological well-being. Using data from integrative medicine, positive psychology, neuropsychiatry, and stress management, we provide a plan that you can use to maintain and support psychological wellness. We also tell you about the latest programs and practices for optimal psychological health including the Neuro Emotional Technique, mindfulness practices, and neurofeedback.

3. *Social*: How many hours a day is your head buried in your laptop or smartphone? Did you know that social connectivity is a hard-wired requirement for optimal brain function? We will discuss the biology of social isolation and all of the important ways of using your social world through family, friends, coworkers, and others. We show you data that support placing importance on maintaining a robust social network for your brain, both in person and online.

4. *Spiritual*: What besides work gives you meaning in life? When you bring ancient and modern spiritual practices into your health management program, healing takes place faster and more often. And we will detail the clinical and brain scan studies that emphasize the transformative results possible from maintaining a strong spiritual or religious component in your life.

Balancing these four dimensions is the best way for you to achieve optimal brain health. In fact, the concept of balance is essential. After all, each ability of the brain typically has a balancing side. Happy emotions have sad emotions, concentration has mind wandering, and excitement has calmness, for example. Each opposite represents an essential function of the brain and each ability of the brain, but if used too much or too little, it can lead to poorer brain health. If we are too happy, we are not realistic, and if we are too sad, we are not open to opportunities. If we concentrate too much, we can miss the forest for the trees, and if we let our mind wander too much, we can become unfocused and unable to complete tasks. The goal is to find the right balance for yourself so that you attain what works best for you and helps you achieve the third perspective on optimal brain health:

#3. Optimal Brain Health = Optimal Brain Balance

This balance applies not just to basic brain functions but to all of the neurophysiology that supports them. Our goal is to help you balance the functioning of the different parts of the brain, the neurotransmitters, and all of the ways in which your brain interacts with the world around you. As the ancient wisdom of the Buddha describes, "If you tighten the string too much, it will snap, and if you leave it too slack, it won't play." The goal is to have the string at just the right balance to allow it to play beautiful music. Similarly, optimal brain health requires finding the right balance to play beautiful music of the mind. We have developed groundbreaking programs in our clinic, and we convey the essence of them in the chapters that follow.

Finally, in order to achieve this ideal of optimal brain health, we ask that instead of blindly and passively assuming that your doctors take care of all aspects of your health, you become empowered coparticipants in directing your brain health behaviors. You can make it happen! From learning to turn on the spiritual circuits in the brain that enhance health, to eating the way ancient sages always recommended and modern science now supports (with some secrets of our own you will learn), you have the ability to engage all of your dimensions and use everything we currently understand to find your own path to optimal brain health.

Chapter 2

IS YOUR BRAIN STARVING TO DEATH? OUR SOLUTION: THE THINK BETTER DIET

The food you eat can either be the safest and most powerful
form of medicine, or the slowest form of poison.

—ANN WIGMORE, 1984

Many people consume an excess of calories and have an excess of body fat, yet at the same time, they are starving their brains. "You are what you eat" is never truer than when referring to the human brain. Are you eating food that energizes and nourishes your brain and body, or food that depletes you and makes you dull, fat, and sick? All of the food you eat ultimately intersects with the hardware of your brain and influences how it functions. In fact, a recent landmark study showed that the plants we eat literally become part of us through a digestive process in which their genomes become incorporated into our own genome.[1]

Does food affect the way we feel emotionally and cognitively? Definitely! But it wasn't that long ago that the psychiatric community scoffed at the notion that food influences psychological states. Some in the community, who are not up on the latest science of food biochemistry, still do. Of course, the relationship makes sense when you think about how many times you may have eaten a piece of chocolate and it made you feel happy, or you binged on junk food and it left you feeling fatigued and depressed. Beyond emotional eating and comfort foods that may have a temporary soothing effect that we later pay for, it is important to continue our concept of self-reflection and pay attention to how food makes our physical bodies feel and how well it makes our brains function. When we do that kind of honest appraisal, we often have to admit to ourselves that some foods we eat—because they are familiar or we think they make us feel comforted in the moment—have a pronounced punishing effect.

We know that food affects short-term inflammation and long-term cognition. In fact, there is an entire gut-brain connection, which we discuss in the next chapter. It is probably already apparent that these relationships have complexities to consider. For example, the occasional "bad food" might be okay, but it is increasingly clear that many of those foods are highly addictive. The junk food industry has food chemists make their products as reinforcing as possible. These calorie-dense, nutrient-poor foods barely deserve the designation as food. For many, they are a poison that gets overconsumed, and for some, they are even the mainstay of their diets. A large study showed a direct correlation of a poor diet to mood/depression in adolescents, and in other studies, diet has been linked to anxiety, lack of concentration, and overall poor cognitive performance.[2] The dietary principles in almost all of the studies point to the same conclusion: our bodies and brains like food—the unadulterated kind that naturally occurs on the planet. Yet overly processed grains, sugars, and animal products define the Western diet, and the evidence is increasingly clear that it is making us sick and dysfunctional.

THE THINK BETTER DIET: THE RIGHT FOOD FOR YOUR BRAIN

Over the past ten years, we have developed at the Marcus Institute the Think Better Diet program based on thousands of research studies, a basic understanding of the human body, and a lot of clinical experience with patients. Some of our conclusions are as much common sense as the good advice your grandmother gave you, while others seem counterintuitive until you understand the science behind them. The integrative brain nutritional approach that we recommend to all of our patients has been shown to help improve brain function and reduce the frequency or symptoms of a number of psychological and neurological diseases.[3]

Although we focus on a number of specific principles in this chapter, there is a continuum of healthful foods that are important to keep in mind as you prepare or order your meals: organic, farm-fresh vegetables are probably the healthiest of all. But if you are going to McDonald's no matter what, we would rather you eat a salad than a hamburger or fried foods. And while fresh vegetables are better than frozen, frozen vegetables are certainly healthier than a lot of prepared and processed foods. As we move down the list, at some point, vegetables can become as unhealthy as other foods. Deep-frying cauliflower and smothering it with cheese products is probably not the best way to go. At that point, you aren't much better off than having fast-food cheese fries. So let us look more specifically at the optimal brain health diet.

The Think Better Diet for optimal brain health has several key components that apply to everyone. From there, it is important to develop your own dietary program based on your likes and dislikes, with the goal of maximizing your brain-body potential. Perhaps the most important point to remember is that you are the one to tailor our integrative diet for your brain and body. We have found that if we meet our patients where they are and then have the goal of getting their diet to the next level, our long-term success is much better than if we take an all-or-nothing approach that is militant and overly restrictive. Of course, there are exceptions. When someone comes to us in a state of illness, we encourage stricter, faster adherence to our diet so as to minimize inflammation in the system and facilitate healing. In our evaluations, we spend a lot of time analyzing what a person eats throughout the day. We do this nonjudgmentally and encourage you to do the same when analyzing your own eating patterns. This isn't about shining the spotlight on how poor your diet is. It is about taking a realistic, self-reflective inventory of the present state of affairs and then making some decisions that will promote a better brain and a better you. Approach this topic as lovingly with yourself as we would with you if you were in front of us for a consultation. Take a moment now to list all the things you typically eat in the course of a day:

Breakfast: _____

Morning snack: _____

Lunch: _____

Midday snack: _____

Dinner: _____

Evening snack: _____

Not only do our dietary recommendations work; most of them have a depth of supportive data. But we need to emphasize that success isn't perfection. It is making meaningful alterations in your diet over time that help you achieve your brain health goals. The first question some of our patients ask, and perhaps you are wondering this too, is how the Think Better Diet will affect your weight. Simply stated, body weight on this program will likely optimize. If you are overweight, you will likely lose those excess pounds—and the more closely you follow the plan, the more you will lose. If you are okay with your weight, you might notice that your body looks different over time and often has a glow and youthfulness that you thought was gone forever. Your skin will look better, and overall you'll exude more energy. All of this is because we are not talking about a short-term diet to lose as much weight as possible. Rather, we are talking about a long-term intervention that, in addition to regulating healthy body weight, will lower systemic inflammation and help your brain and body thrive. As you take a deeper dive into your diet, be patient but tenacious. We have four key principles to keep in mind:

1. *Plants feed your brain.* The best evidence to date suggests that a plant-based diet is the healthiest for your brain.[4] Green leafy plants are especially packed with phytonutrients—nutritional molecules found in plants—and it is best to aim for at least two servings of them a day—raw and fresh whenever possible. These are the life and energy of your diet.

2. *Processed foods starve your brain.* In fact, in many cases, they also harm your brain. Grains come from a plant, but the reality is that the majority of grains we have access to are highly processed. It is also essential to eat the most natural foods, reduce simple carbohydrates found in starches and sugars, and eliminate processed foods and red meat.

3. *Healthy fats protect your brain.* The third goal of your diet is to increase the amount of healthy fats you consume since they are good for your brain.[5] The Think Better Diet encourages you to make sure you are getting some nuts, seeds, and olive oil in your diet every day.

4. *Unhealthy fats destroy your brain.* Animal fats, except fresh fish, and processed vegetable oils increase inflammation in the body.[6] It is important to use lean and plant-based protein sources in place of animal products that have high amounts of destructive animal fat, such as luncheon meats and dairy.

Let's break these down in more detail. The first point is to eat a more plant-based diet. Of all the living things on the earth, plants are the only ones that directly convert the sun's energy into biological energy. In some sense, when you eat a plant, you are eating sunshine, and the sun is what gives energy to all life on earth.

So why not get your energy as directly as possible from the sun? Eating plants is the best way to do that. Our general rule is that if it grows, it's good for you!

Vegetables, fruits, nuts, seeds, and legumes comprise virtually all of the plant-based foods. An important point is that there are lots of options out there when it comes to eating plant-based foods. Just because you don't like broccoli or Brussels sprouts doesn't mean you can't find a wide range of other plant foods to enjoy. Please see our listing of a wide variety of common plant foods on pages 31–34. We hope that somewhere on this list, you can find several choices that you really enjoy and be open to experimenting with others to widen the range of your palate. If there are some that you have never tried, now is the time.

We also emphasize that there are lots of delicious options for preparing these foods, some of which you may have never considered. You don't just have to eat salad all the time to achieve the overarching goal of dramatically increasing the amount of vegetables and plant-based foods you eat. We like to use as a starting goal doubling the amount of whichever ones you are eating now during the next week. Think about increasing vegetables at snack time by dipping them into guacamole, hummus, or whatever else your favorite plant-based spread is. You can roast the these vegetables in the oven with garlic and oregano. You can make a stir-fry or roll them in a wrap. Make sure you explore lots of different options and ways of spicing up these vegetables so that you can enjoy them in as many ways as possible. And of course, they make wonderful side dishes for whatever other foods you might eat. If you are at a restaurant, ask for an extra helping of vegetables instead of bread, pasta, or potatoes.

An important point about plant-based foods is that there are now many options with high-protein content. Getting more of the proteins you eat from plants is an essential part of the success of the Think Better Diet. This is supported by excellent studies that show plant-based proteins are much healthier than animal-based ones, particularly in terms of overall health risks.[7] Good sources of plant-based proteins are legumes and beans, including lentils and chickpeas, as well as soy-based foods such as tofu in moderation. It is helpful to try and work as many of these plant-based protein sources into your nutrition throughout the day.

In addition to eating natural plant foods, we often encourage our patients to use plant-based protein and meal replacement shakes to ensure sufficient plant protein and also to have as standbys when they aren't sure what to eat at a given meal or as a midday snack. Several companies make these shakes with numerous flavor options. To see which ones we use at the Marcus Institute, visit our website at marcusinstitute.jeffersonhealth.org and click on "Shop." The website also has great information and updates, our faculty blog posts on the latest information in the field, and more. (This is a service the institute provides and we do not personally financially benefit from product sales.) If you want to explore other potential shakes, we recommend those with plant-based proteins such as pea protein. We also recommend shakes that are low in carbohydrates—less than 10 grams—and high in proteins and good fats.

These shakes can be mixed with water or with your favorite milk alternative like almond or oat milk, which give them a creamier texture. They mix well with no need to use any equipment if you want something quick and easy, and they are easy to take on the go; just put the powder in a bottle before you leave, add water, and shake when you are ready to drink it. These shakes are loaded with good proteins, vitamins, and nutrients, and they are low in simple carbs. We frequently recommend them to replace a meal such as a typical breakfast or a midday snack. This can be particularly helpful if your usual breakfast is a starchy muffin or bagel, or nothing at all. Another great option for these shakes is to put them in a blender with some ice and a handful of mild greens like spinach. You will be amazed at how delicious they make a vegetable taste, and you now have the double whammy of a healthy meal with living nutrients. Some people add a little almond butter to their chocolate drink as well to give it a rich texture. Others add natural flavor extracts such as vanilla or cinnamon.

Nuts and seeds have protein and satisfy another key healthy diet concept: good fats that help reduce inflammation in the brain and body and aid in building cell membranes and supporting essential cellular functions.[8] Please see page 33 for a list of healthy nuts and seeds. These can make great snacks or can be used in various meals. For example, you might consider almond-crusted salmon or put walnuts or pumpkin seeds in a salad. Note that peanuts are technically a legume and do not have the same health benefits. In fact, their fat is of the inflammatory type so it is best to replace your peanut butter with almond butter, cashew butter, or something similar.

A critical key concept is to minimize processed foods, which also offers an opportunity to maximize your use of more whole grains. The "whole grain" label refers to a grain in which all components of the grain—the bran, germ, and endosperm—remain intact. A grain can be considered "whole" whether it is in its more natural state or is ground into flour. One of the main reasons whole grains are better than processed grains is they contain more fiber, which has been shown to reduce blood pressure and the buildup of plaque (atherosclerosis) in arteries.[9] Reducing these risks also helps protect the brain by maintaining appropriate blood flow for its functions. In addition, fiber in many cases feeds the healthy bacteria in the gut microbiome and acts as a "prebiotic" or a nutrient that supports the growth of good bacteria. More to come on the microbiome in the next chapter.

When selecting foods, think about avoiding those that come in boxes and cans. For the most part, these contain high levels of salt, processed oils, and other chemicals and preservatives, all of which can adversely affect the brain.[10] And sometimes the containers themselves have chemicals that impair biological processes.[11]

While we strongly encourage plant-based foods, a healthful diet can also consist of lean meats such as turkey, chicken, and various fishes. The best fish to consider are salmon, tuna, and sardines since they have a high oil content—"good" oils that reduce inflammation and provide essential fats for brain function. Other good fish include mackerel, perch, rainbow trout, striped bass, wild Alaskan pollock, and arctic char.

If you are going to incorporate fish or some meat in your diet, it is important to try to eat animal-based ones that are as natural and organic as possible and as little processed as possible. Highly processed meats such as bacon, hotdogs, and scrapple have many chemicals in them that are toxic for your brain and body. Studies have demonstrated that higher intakes of all of these highly processed meats result in increased all-cause mortality.[12] But if you have no choice other than to eat some type of processed food, at least try to find options that have reduced salt, no added sugars, or no high-fructose corn syrup; are made with good oils such as olive oil; and are low in saturated and trans fats.

Another common concern with many of these foods is that those that are the healthiest are often the most expensive. Buying organic or farm-fresh foods can be two to four times more expensive than regular. For those on a limited budget, there are many helpful alternatives that while not necessarily as good as organics are still far healthier than highly processed foods and meats. For example, raw vegetables that are not organic are still healthier than highly processed foods, and plant foods with thick skins like melons, oranges, squash, and zucchini can be easily peeled and cleansed of any pesticides and chemicals that might be on them.[13] Even frozen vegetables are usually better than processed foods. And adding in beans and legumes can be an excellent source of proteins that are low in cost and easy to prepare.

CONSTRUCTING THE THINK BETTER DIET

With these general principles in mind, let's review the basic ideas behind the Think Better Diet to help you construct a brain-healthy diet:

Principles for Success

- *Practice mindful eating.* Think about everything you put in your body and ask yourself if it's a "giver" or a "taker." Do not eat while watching television or doing other things. Eat in a relaxed environment, and be sure to chew each mouthful five to ten times to help break down the food even before it gets to your stomach, thus making it easier to digest.

- *Drink five to eight glasses of water a day.* If you are hydrated, you will be less hungry and healthier. The brain needs sufficient hydration for optimal performance.

- *Avoid all regular and diet soft drinks.* Avoid soda and other drinks that have artificial colors and sweeteners, especially aspartame. The sweetener in regular soda is as brain unhealthy as it gets. Choose unsweetened herbal teas, kombucha drinks, and naturally flavored waters instead.

- *Eat breakfast every day.* It is critical to eat breakfast, but in a different way than you are probably used to. Morning is a great time to have some vegetable protein, such as a hemp shake, or to use your rice cooker or steamer to prepare a variety of fresh grains.

- *Listen to your gut.* If a food makes you feel badly, it probably is bad for you! Take note of how certain foods make you feel after you eat them.

- *Bring one to two healthful snacks to work or school.* Raw vegetables, raw almonds or walnuts, and plant-alternative yogurt such as from soy, almond, or rice are great examples of these snacks.

- *Dark, fresh fruits are best.* Generally a brain-healthy integrative diet encourages you to eat up to two servings of dark, fleshy fruit every day as a snack or treat. Good fruits include plums and berries. Avoid commercial bananas, most grapes, and dried fruits because they contain a lot of sugar.

- *Eat whole, unprocessed grains.* Avoid refined, polished, and processed foods such as pasta, rice, bread, crackers, and snack foods.

- *Limit animal fat and protein.* The best form of animal protein is fresh, wild fish—up to three servings per week. Fish also has the added bonus of healthy fat. Red meats—beef, pork, and lamb, to name a few—are best to avoid, but *occasional* organic, free-range poultry eggs—one serving per week—is okay. Commercial meats and poultry are often highly contaminated with problematic chemicals. Dairy milk and dairy milk products are discouraged at all times.

- *Avoid trans fat altogether.* Fortunately, trans fats have been banned in most foods, but they still surface in margarine, fried foods, baked goods, and processed, ready-to-serve foods.

- *Eat "healthy" fat.* Fatty fish, like salmon, as well as the fats in plant-based foods like flaxseeds, avocados, nuts, and vegetable oils such as olive and canola, and nut and seed oils like sesame and sunflower, are good choices.

- *Plant-based protein is a key to success.* Contrary to popular belief, many plants provide excellent sources of protein. Specifically, legumes (beans), soy, and whole grains can provide all the protein you need to build muscle and lose fat. We also recommend hemp protein powder for those who want some supplemental protein.

- *Clean your vegetables and fruits thoroughly.* Make sure to wash all unpackaged produce such as leafy greens and even prewashed pro-duce like bagged spinach under running water prior to meal prepa-ration. Consider using a salad spinner for easy washing.

- *Spice up your diet.* Many delicious spices, such as dried red pepper, chili peppers, and rosemary, show some ability to reduce hunger, improve mood and brainpower, and even help muscles stay strong.

- *Go NUTS.* Studies show that some types of nuts, particularly wal-nuts, can have a positive impact on cardiovascular health. However, avoid peanuts: they are a legume, and their fat is not healthy.

- *Use olive oil.* Cold-pressed, extra-virgin olive oil is the preferred oil for salads and cooking. Just add lemon and fresh herbs to make a delicious dressing. Olive oil is rich in polyphenols, an important plant nutrient, and is anti-inflammatory.

- *Eat more veggies!* As counterintuitive as this might seem, when you swap out processed foods for fresh veggies, you need to increase the volume of food you are eating. If you were to put the food you currently eat each day on a scale, it might weigh four to five pounds, which is average. You need a certain amount of bulk and weight going through your gastrointestinal (GI) track to keep it healthy. When you eat four pounds of vegetable foods, that amounts to a much higher volume than if you were eating four pounds of processed foods, because processed foods tend to be much more calorically and physically dense—they are similar weights but very different calories. A half-pound of pepperoni pizza is much more calorie-dense than half a pound of arugula.

FOODS TO INCLUDE IN AN INTEGRATIVE DIET

PROTEINS

Beans and legumes: Eat lentils, chickpeas, adzuki beans, and other legumes and beans only in amounts that you can digest well. If you find that these are upsetting your stomach with gas, bloating, constipation, or diarrhea, reduce the amount and frequency.

Fresh fish: Wild fish is better than farm-raised, with a limit of three servings of fish per week.

Plant-based products: Tempeh, mushroom burgers, and tofu are fine, but avoid seitan because of the gluten, which many people can have a sensitivity to.

Vegan protein powder: Mix these powders derived from soy, pea, or hemp with a low-sugar, nondairy milk alternative such as almond milk.

VEGETABLES

Greens:

Bok choy	Lettuce
Cabbage	Mustard greens
Chinese cabbage	Parsley
Collard greens	Spinach
Endive	Swiss chard
Escarole	Watercress
Kale	

Other Great Vegetable/Vegetable-Like Options

Alfalfa sprouts	Onions
Artichoke hearts	Pumpkin
Asparagus	Radishes
Avocado	Scallions
Bean sprouts	Shallots
Broccoli	Snow peas
Broccoli rabe	Squash
Brussels sprouts	String/Green beans
Cauliflower	Turnips
Celery	Zucchini
Cucumber	
Mushrooms	
(shiitake, portobello,	
crimini, white)	

We typically recommend avoiding nightshade vegetables such as white potatoes, tomatoes, eggplant, and bell peppers since they can be inflammatory and can contain a variety of poisonous compounds, although usually in low amounts. We also recommend limiting higher-carb veggies such as carrots, yams, and squash to two to three servings per week and eating fresh sprouts several times a week

GRAINS

Amaranth	Millet
Barley	Quinoa
Brown rice	Rye
Buckwheat (kasha)	

Quinoa is more of a seed than a grain and is one of our favorite food options. It cooks well, has high nutritional value, and is gluten free. We recommend completely avoiding wheat and oats by those who are gluten sensitive, though gluten-free oats can be okay in moderation. Those who have any food sensitivities should avoid corn entirely.

NUTS AND SEEDS

Raw nuts and seeds are by far the preferred variety, particularly walnuts, almonds, and pumpkin seeds. Other good raw choices are sunflower seeds, pine nuts, flax seeds, and chia seeds. Chia is an ancient food dating back thousands of years to the Aztecs and has a high nutritional value, but is relatively new in the modern Western world. When you can't get nuts and seeds raw, roasted ones with light or no salt added are still far better than snacking on potato chips. Cashews, macadamia nuts, and others high in fat are best in moderation

Almonds	Pecans
Brazil nuts	Pine nuts
Cashews	Pumpkin seeds
Flaxseeds	Sesame seeds
(ground is better	Sunflower seeds
than whole)	Walnuts
Macadamia nuts	

FRUITS

This is a list of fruits with the best antioxidant benefits that are also among the lowest in sugar. Citrus fruits, such as oranges and grapefruit, are okay in moderation. Some fruits, such as bananas and many other varieties of grapes besides red grapes, have high sugar content, which is why they don't appear on this list.

Blueberries

Cherries

Plums

Raspberries

Red grapes

(no more than

10 per serving)

SNACKS

The best snacks are vegetables, vegetable protein shakes, healthy trail mix low in sugar and saturated fats, soy yogurt, whole grain crackers (Mary's Gone Crackers and Ryvita are preferred brands), and 100 percent buckwheat crackers. For those trying to limit calories, apples can be a good snack because they are filling and have high fiber—but enjoy them on their own without combining with other foods and eat no more than two a day.

We recommend these spreads and dips:

Almond butter

Guacamole

Hummus

Pesto

Tahini

Tofu spread

DRINKS

Green tea

Herbal tea

Spring or

filtered water

PROTEIN SHAKE BRANDS

Plant Fusion   Vega One

OTHER DIET PROGRAMS

While we recommend our Think Better Diet because it is built on the best evidence-based medicine to date, there are certainly many other types of diets out there. The problem is that there are too many different programs, and it is difficult to know what to make of all of them. Some, in particular, don't sound particularly healthy such as the Candy Diet and the Cookie Diet. We found the following ones that sound dubious and probably still missed a bunch:

3 Day Diet	Dean Ornish Diet	Metabolism Diet
Abs Diet	Eat Subway and	Miracle Diet
Acai Berry Diet	Lose Weight	Negative Calorie Diet
Apple Cider	Fruit Diet	Paleo Diet
Vinegar Diet	Grapefruit Juice	Peanut Butter Diet
Atkin's Diet	Diet	Popcorn Diet
Beverly Hills Diet	HCG Diet	Potato Chips Diet
Blood Type Diet	Ice Cream Diet	Pritikin Diet
Brazilian Diet	Intermittent Fasting	Sacred Heart Diet
Cabbage Soup Diet	Keto Diet	Salad Diet
Candy Diet	Lemonade Diet	Scarsdale Diet
Chicken Soup Diet	Liquid Diet	Soup Diet
Chocolate Diet	Low-Carb Diet	South Beach Diet
Coconut Diet	Low-Fat Diet	Three Apples
Coffee Diet	Maple Syrup Diet	a Day Diet
Cookie Diet	Master Cleanse Diet	Tuna Diet
Dash Diet	Mediterranean Diet	Zone Diet

The most important thing to know about these diets is what foods they use and, perhaps more important, how the macronutrients—protein, carbohydrates, and fats—are proportioned. The overarching goal of most of these diets is to lose weight. As a general rule, diets typically restrict one type of macronutrient in a prominent way. So the Ornish Diet, for example, is low fat with a moderate amount of carbohydrates and proteins. At the opposite end of the spectrum is the Atkin's Diet, which is low in carbohydrates and high in fats and proteins.

In terms of the Think Better Diet, the focus is on what will maximize your personal performance. Your trimness will take care of itself if you follow our simple guidelines, with optimal body weight being one of the many bonuses of the program versus a singular focus. Maintaining a healthy body weight is important for optimal brain health, and losing weight can lead to lower blood pressure, insulin resistance, cholesterol levels, and risk of development of atherosclerosis.

AN IMPORTANT FINAL NOTE

Sugar is the great destroyer along with its accomplices, bad fat and toxic chemicals. We all know that sugar is the white stuff in packets or in a sugar bowl, but it also comes in many other forms, such as high-fructose corn syrup—the common sweetener in soda and other beverages—as well as being quickly created in the gut by eating simple starches such as white bread and white rice. The excessive sugar load that Americans consume from these sources is destroying our brains and bodies, causing insulin resistance, neurological instability, and toxic inflammation.[14] Many people are addicted to the taste of sweetness, and it will take some patience and self-kindness to get past it. But if you eat enough of the foods we suggest so that you are not hungry, your cravings for sweets will diminish. Also, drink plenty of water and other low-sugar beverages such as brewed herbal teas. Hydration is important for your brain health and for helping to combat cravings. By following these guidelines, you will provide your brain with the nutrients and energy it needs while reducing the amount of harmful substances that can impair your brain's functions or, worse, damage the only brain you will ever have.

Chapter 3

YOUR GUT HEALTH CAN DETERMINE YOUR BRAIN HEALTH

All disease begins in the gut.

—Hippocrates, circa 400 BC

We've all heard of the mind-body connection. Some of the latest science on this large topic is centered around the fascinating connections between gut and brain. It makes sense when you think about it. As we discussed in the previous chapter, your brain health relies heavily on what you eat; hence, the overall health and functionality of your gut—how it processes nutrients and protects you from the outside environment—must be an important factor. But what exactly is gut health, and how does that have anything to do with your diet and nutrition? Certainly the health of your gut is determined in large part by what you eat. But there are other important gut considerations that you need to know about for optimal brain health.

THE GUT MICROBIOME

The amount and types of bacteria in your gut, known as the *gut microbiome*, are essential for maintaining good health. Ask yourself how many cells you think are in the average human body. The answer is about 30 trillion, give or take. How many bacteria do we host in our bodies? The answer is the same, and it may even be slightly more. Most of these bacteria live in the gut, and their influence is profound. While these are much smaller cells—weighing in total only a couple of pounds—they have tremendous genetic content that can influence your overall health. There can be thousands of species in your gut at any time, and the balance of those species means everything. Some are good, and some are not so good, so the ratio of good to bad is critical.

If you have the right balance of bacteria, your gut and brain will stay optimally healthy. And if you have the wrong bacteria, your gut and brain can suffer from a variety of illnesses. There have even been some fascinating studies in animals, and recently in humans, that show that the types of bacteria in your gut is directly connected to what is going on in your brain. One study looked at mice that expressed behaviors as if they were depressed; for example, they didn't play with their new toys and or engage with other mice.[1] But when these mice that acted depressed were given a fecal transplant (the poop from another mouse) from a nondepressed mouse, their symptoms improved. Similarly, normal mice that were given a fecal transplant from a depressed mouse began to demonstrate behaviors of depression. The main point of this study was that the bacteria in the feces of the depressed- and nondepressed-acting mice seemed to be essential to how they behaved. Thus, the bacteria in your gut might be one of the most important factors affecting your mood—maybe even more than all of the bad things that happen in life.

Researchers are beginning to explore whether such an approach might be viable in human beings as well. While the concept might seem a bit off-putting, it is fundamentally important for our discussion about how gut health and brain health are linked. The good news is that you can do things that have a positive impact on the balance of bacteria in your gut. How to maintain a good bacterial milieu in the gut requires much of what this book is about, especially the Think Better Diet plan. There are relatively few people who are blessed with exceptionally good genes and gut bacteria that keep everything working smoothly, even when they don't follow our guidelines. These outliers are able to eat lots of different foods without having any problems with gas, bloating, or a change in bowel habits. Furthermore, foods that these people eat do not have an impact on their mood or cognition.

But for many, and really most, people, eating the wrong foods can create all kinds of symptoms, both physical and mental. These symptoms, combined with other factors that alter gut health, like chronic stress and exposure to toxins, can lead to a needlessly unhappy life. We have already seen that working toward a plant-based, protein-based, anti-inflammatory diet is a great way to start weaving a healthier brain. While we believe there is no substitute for eating a diet high in plant fibers that feeds the good gut bacteria, the data so far that supplementing with bacteria in the form of probiotics is highly useful in balancing the microbiome of the gut are limited.[2] For example, one study showed that patients with major depression who took a daily probiotic combination of *Lactobacillus acidophilus, Lactobacillus casei,* and *Bifidobacterium bifidum* for eight weeks had significant improvements in their depression scores.[3] These additions also improved the body's metabolism, inflammation levels in the body as measured by C-reactive protein concentrations, and antioxidant status as measured by higher levels of glutathione. This study shows that many body processes are reflected in how well the brain operates and that those processes can be improved with probiotics.

GUT HEALTH AND INFLAMMATION

Let's look at how all of this fits together. The gut regulates inflammation and brings in nutrients to the body, and the brain depends on those nutrients but also reacts negatively to excess inflammatory chemicals. (*Inflammation* is a generic term that refers to the body's response to insult and injury.) Externally we think about the hallmarks of inflammation as pain, redness, and swelling. But the chemical processes behind those musculoskeletal injuries are also going on inside the body to address internal imbalances, such as when pathogens along the gut wall cause destruction. The "good" bacteria protect us from these. In addition, foods can cause a release of those inflammatory chemicals such as ones from saturated animal fat and processed foods, whereas foods such as leafy greens and omega-3 essential fat from fish and plants have an anti-inflammatory effect. Also, healthy food promotes healthy bacteria by providing an environment it needs in order to thrive.

Perturbations of the gut microbiota, referred to as *gut dysbiosis*, are commonly described in many diseases involving inflammation. The reason is that the gut has an entire immune system all to itself: the gut-associated lymphoid tissue or GALT. These immune cells watch everything that is happening in the gut. If the gut is invaded by the wrong bacteria, the GALT sends immune signals throughout the body, causing systemic inflammation. Imagine how you feel when you are sick. The same feeling arises when your gut has the wrong bacteria. There is also a vicious cycle that occurs because the inflamed microenvironment in the gut is particularly conducive to a proliferation of bad bacteria such as *Enterobacteriaceae*, while families of potentially healthful bacteria such as *Lactobacillales* succumb to those same environmental changes.[4]

The gut microbiome accounts for about 1 to 3 percent of your total body mass.[5] More important than absolute cell numbers is that the total bacterial genes outnumber human genes by about 150:1, and more than ten thousand different species may reside in the microbiome. The human genome has twenty-three thousand genes, but the microbiome has over 1 million genes. The potential impact of the microbiome is clearly huge, so it stands to reason that taking care of your microbiome is essential for weaving a healthy brain. But how do you best take care of your gut microbiome, especially when you can't see it?

MAINTAINING A HEALTHY GUT

One of the ways we like to help our patients think about keeping a healthy gut microbiome is by using the analogy of having a really good grass lawn. The best way to have a healthy lawn is to have a strong natural turf with a variety of good types of grass that are hearty and full. When you have a thick natural turf, weeds cannot grow easily because they are squeezed out by the naturally good grass; in addition, the soil itself stays healthy. In a similar way, a full and thick healthy gut microbiome largely prevents bad bacteria from growing and keeps inflammation of the gut itself to a minimum. The best way to manage this naturally is by eating the right foods and avoiding the bad ones through the Think Better Diet program.

But sometimes there is damage to the turf. It could be from drought or from not getting enough nutrients. In a similar way, the gut microbiome can be damaged by an infection, the use of certain medications—particularly antibiotics—or just poor diet. If some of that good turf begins to weaken, weeds can take root and grow. If there are just a few patches of weeds, the turf itself may still be pretty healthy. Sometimes you can help these weak areas by throwing down some good seed. In many ways, using a probiotic is like that. The probiotic has the "seeds" of good bacteria—actually the bacteria—that can help overcome many bad patches in the microbiome. But sometimes just spreading seed is not good enough, and you have to make sure that you put the right amount of fertilizer on to provide the right nutrients so that the natural turf can grow well. Fertilizer for the gut comes in the form of prebiotics and a healthy diet, both of which contain the nutrients the good bacteria need in order to flourish.

If the patches of weeds become too great, sometimes you need to put weed killer down. In terms of the gut, this sometimes takes the form of various foods or natural supplements that can inhibit bad bacteria and allow the good bacteria to grow. And in a worst-case scenario, sometimes you have to dig up all of the grass and start completely over. In integrative medicine, sometimes we treat people who fit this description with a strong antibiotic such as rifamixin that will kill most of the bacteria, both good and bad, but more selectively the bad. Then we add the seeds of good bacteria using probiotics and fertilize with prebiotics.

We hope that this garden analogy helps you understand a bit more about how good bacteria work and how to take care of your gut. (For more information about products we recommend, visit our website at marcusinstitute.jefferson-health.org, and be sure to sign up for our free newsletter for the latest updates on the microbiome and much more.)

Let's now take a deeper dive into the science of the gut microbiome and its effects on human health:

Microbiome (Who's there?): The composite of commensal, symbiotic, and pathogenic microbial species that are living in the gut. There are numerous emerging technologies and techniques to assess the content and health of the microenvironment of the gut.

Metagenomics (What language do they speak?): Genomic analysis of microbial DNA that is extracted directly from communities in environmental samples. This technology—genomics on a large scale—enables a survey of the microorganisms present in the gut environment.

Metascriptomics (What are they talking about?): Proteins and other signaling molecules of a group of interacting organisms or species. This technique enables identifying the actively transcribed ribosomal and messenger RNA from a community of bacteria in the microbiome.

In terms of the microbiome itself, the two largest types of bacteria are called Firmicutes and Bacteroidetes. An altered relationship in the Firmicutes-to-Bacteroidetes ratio has been associated with a number of pathological conditions. For example, obesity has been associated with an increased abundance of Firmicutes, a decrease in Bacteroidetes, or both.[6] This ratio is also related to a disruption of metabolic homeostasis that can lead to diabetes or nonalcoholic fatty liver disease and elevated markers of inflammation.[7] The balance is also important for brain health. Studies have shown that Bacteroidetes are increased and Firmicutes decreased in patients with depression.[8] But more important, one study using mice showed that when the gut microbiome shifted to a depression-inducing pattern, activity in the hippocampus changed.[9] Since the hippocampus is part of the limbic system and intimately involved in depression, this overall relationship drives home the point that the microbiome can deeply affect the brain. In addition, the hippocampus is responsible for processing long-term memory, storage of long-term memories, and memory of the location of objects or people. Protecting the hippocampus therefore helps not only with depression but with cognition as well.

In another recent study, prebiotics were shown to have anxiolytic and antidepressant-like effects and to reverse the impact of chronic stress in mice.[10] And a growing number of studies in humans have shown how probiotics can reduce anxiety symptoms in both healthy people and those in certain patient populations. These findings are important. If probiotics can help reduce anxiety in healthy people, they can be useful in general for protecting against stress and anxiety. In other words, they can help you weave together a stronger brain that is resistant to external stressors. And if you have a condition such as irritable bowel syndrome (IBS), chronic fatigue syndrome, or cancer, the research shows that probiotics might even be useful for reducing the associated higher levels of anxiety—clearly a much better way than taking a benzodiazepine like Xanax or Valium.

Changes in the gut microbiome might also contribute to changes in cognition. Studies have shown that supplementation with probiotics can greatly influence brain function, including increased neuroplasticity—the ability of neurons to grow and sprout new connections. This neuroplasticity is essential for obtaining and maintaining high levels of cognitive function.

The gut microbiome also influences cognitive function via the gut-brain axis and helps maintain the integrity of the blood-brain barrier, which helps protect the brain from toxins and other insults, meaning that maintaining a good barrier supports a healthy brain. But the blood-brain barrier does not fare as well when people eat a typical Western diet, particularly high-fat and high-sugar diets that increase Firmicutes and decrease Bacteroidetes.[11]

If you are thinking about taking a probiotic, it is important to consider how healthy your gut may already by answering these questions:

1. Do you have chronic gastrointestinal symptoms such as reflux, gas and bloating, or diarrhea and constipation?

2. Do any members in your family exhibit similar kinds of symptoms with their gastrointestinal tract?

3. Have you noticed any correlations between the food you eat and your overall brain function in terms of cognition and mood?

This third question can be difficult to answer at times, but it might be helpful to think back as to whether your moods change around different times of the week, such as after weekend splurges on food or alcohol or after consuming certain types of foods such as those with lots of carbohydrates. If you have answered yes to any of these questions, you might consider having your gut tested for the different types of bacteria. This can help provide an understanding of the overall balance of bacteria in your gut and help you determine whether a rebalancing would contribute to your overall brain health. Gut-testing kits can help you determine which bacteria you have, which ones you need, and which ones you have but don't want. Your doctor can prescribe the test that is best for you.

Some have even argued that everyone would be better off by taking a probiotic to help maintain their bacterial system and also protect against future insults such as from infections, the use of antibiotics, the use of other medications, or the need for different surgical procedures. Others argue that there aren't enough data from clinical trials to make this a universal recommendation. We help our patients arrive at the decision that is best for them based on the health of their gut. However, we always use probiotics in an integrated plan that includes dietary interventions.

Currently available probiotics fall into several categories based on the type of bacteria they contain. A large number of probiotics contain Lactobacillus or Bifidobacteria species, or both. These are the most common "good" bacteria in the gut. Studies have shown Lactobacillus to be helpful against yeast infections, bacterial vaginosis, urinary tract infections, and diarrhea related to antibiotic use, traveler's diarrhea, or *Clostridium difficile*. Bifidobacteria have been found to be helpful in patients with IBS. The amount each person needs can vary, just as long as it is enough to get through the stomach. We typically recommend 50 billion to 100 billion colony-forming units (CFUs).

Another type of probiotic contains *Saccharomyces boulardii*, a healthy yeast for the gut. It is believed to be particularly good for preventing diarrhea, including infectious types such as viral diarrhea, diarrhea caused by bacterial overgrowth of "bad" bacteria in the gut, and traveler's diarrhea. Other people use *S. boulardii* for lactose intolerance, vaginal yeast infections, and urinary tract infections.

Two important factors to consider when choosing a probiotic are how many bacteria they deliver and whether they are shelf-stable. This means that you ideally want your probiotic to not require refrigeration since many can lose potency fast, even during delivery transit or while sitting on a store shelf. Ideally you want your probiotic to have a shelf life of two years. It is also important probiotics to have a relatively high CFU count (at least 50 billion per serving). Probiotics that have low CFU counts, especially when contained in foods like yogurt, are typically not effective. Going back to the lawn analogy, it is like throwing a handful of seeds onto a large area of soil—not enough to have any effect. Similarly, it is helpful to find probiotics that have a delayed-release mechanism that protects the probiotics from stomach acid and allows more of them to get into the intestines where they are needed.

A stool study will help identify more precisely what bacteria you may need. But if you want to take a probiotic without a lot of diagnostic testing, it is probably best to select one that has a good diversity of friendly bacteria. For instance, a probiotic that has six or more bacterial strains, including Bacillus and Lactobacillus strains, is more likely to help your gut find a good balance.

And finishing with our lawn analogy, it can be helpful to find a product that has both probiotics and prebiotics, which is like getting grass seed already combined with a fertilizer. The prebiotic provides the nutrients to support the growth of the probiotics once they get into your system. Sufficient prebiotics often are found in a healthy diet that incorporates enough plant fiber, though we also recommend using prebiotic products in many cases.

In the end, no matter how much testing you do or which probiotic you choose, be careful to watch for downsides as well as benefits. It is always important to involve your doctors in these plans. And if your bowel habits change, such as the onset of diarrhea or abdominal discomfort, stop and consider another plan. It is equally important to determine if your plan is providing a benefit. Do you feel better? Does your gut feel happier? Do you feel happier? Using a probiotic can be a fundamental part in weaving together a tapestry of optimal brain health.

Chapter 4

PREVENTING A TOXIC BRAIN

Look after your brain.

W. Richie Russell, 1975

O ver your lifetime, you are exposed to hundreds, if not thousands, of toxins in the environment. Many have been around long before human beings even showed up on the planet. Volcanoes, for instance, spew out all kinds of chemicals and heavy metals that can be incorporated into plant and animal life. Radioactive materials abound in nature and can cause various types of mutations and injure cellular processes. Even oxygen itself, essential for life, can be highly injurious if the wrong forms of it are excessive in our biochemistry. Referred to as reactive oxygen species (ROS), injuries from this form of oxygen, known as oxidative stress or oxidative damage, are observed in and are at the root cause of a variety of human illnesses, including many neurodegenerative diseases. We will get more into ROS injuries and how to minimize them later in the chapter.

With the industrial production of so many new types of molecules and chemicals, we see toxins of all types invading our environment, confusing our biology, and contributing to disease. Toxins can also be in the form of various metals that influence cellular processes or act as catalysts for different reactions in the body and brain. Toxic plastics and related compounds can also find their way into a variety of animals that humans consume. In particular, antibiotics are used excessively in the livestock industry to ward off infections from the poor living conditions of the animals and also to make them grow larger and produce more meat.

The problem is that those antibiotics get into our gut when we consume the meat, resulting in a disruption to our entire physiology, including contributing to antibiotic resistance. Pesticides and other compounds are sprayed into the air to protect plants, but they also seep into the ground and water. From there they accumulate in our systems, and the toxicity profiles of many aren't encouraging. If you took a blood test right now, you would likely have more than thirty of these pesticide chemicals in your bloodstream.[1] Finally, synthetic hormones are used to help animals grow larger, produce more milk, and feed more people. These hormones can also have a negative impact on the body and brain.

This information can seem a bit overwhelming and even doomsday sounding; however, it is still good to be aware of your exposure to toxins even if you think your risk is low. And the good news is that your brain and body are built with incredible resiliency, as well as checks and balances to navigate the toxic storm we are all continuously exposed to and therefore are able to withstand a substantial amount of toxic insult. Your metabolic system, including the liver and kidneys, immune system, and antioxidant system, all enable your body to eliminate or reduce the toxic burden on it so you can stay alive.

The bad news is that often we are unknowingly overwhelming the delicate checks and balances of the brain and body to deal with those toxins. And if the toxic burden becomes too great, disease and dysfunction begin to occur. What is also interesting is that we each have different abilities to deal with toxins. For example, we could line up ten people who are full of mercury, and seven of them will feel completely fine. Two of them may end up with cancer as the result of their exposure to mercury, and one of them may be highly symptomatic with all kinds of muscular, neurological, and physiological problems. So it is essential to not only understand what toxins are but also, and more important, how to minimize your exposure and decrease your personal toxic burden.

This type of exposure has been linked to a number of conditions. Chronic pain, chronic fatigue, cognitive and emotional dysfunction, cancer, cardiovascular disease, immunological disorders, and rheumatological disorders have all been associated with various toxins. Some of these are clearly related to specific toxic compounds. For example, the famous Mad Hatter in Lewis Carroll's *Alice's Adventures in Wonderland* was based on actual people back in the 1800s who made hats and had chronic exposure to mercury in their work process. Chronic exposure to mercury can lead to serious psychiatric disorders.

Another specific toxic effect is associated with a molecule called MPTP (the acronym for the long chemical name: 1-methyl-4-phenyl-1,2,3,6-tetrahydropyridine). Originally this substance was accidentally produced when people were trying to make synthetic opioids in the 1970s. Instead, they made MPTP, which turned out to be a molecule that is extremely detrimental to the dopamine neurons in the brain and the result is an acute development of Parkinson's syndrome which appears with all the symptoms of Parkinson's but is not technically Parkinson's disease—a neurodegenerative process that occurs in older individuals.[2] Unfortunately, many of these individuals from the seventies expressed all of the symptoms and disabilities associated with Parkinson's disease, an incurable condition. However, if there is a positive side to this, MPTP has been used over the years as a research model for Parkinson's, particularly in animal studies, as a way to help develop drugs that can protect people from the development of the disease.

So the question we have to address is how best to deal with toxins if we want to maintain an optimal brain. After all, we don't want to muck up the delicate weave we are trying to create within the neuronal connections of the brain. Part of the answer to this question, as we consider throughout this book, is, "What are your own personal strengths and vulnerabilities when it comes to toxins?"

Several genetic tests give a sense as to whether your body can handle various toxins and to what extent. A variety of enzymes, many of them in your liver, can have their genetics explored to determine whether you are a fast or slow metabolizer of different compounds. For example, some people have a great deal of alcohol dehydrogenase and are thus able to handle alcohol, as a toxin, to a much greater degree than others. Those who do not have significant alcohol dehydrogenase in the liver, or a mutated version, can be highly susceptible to the toxic effects of alcohol. These individuals can even die from exposure to excessive alcohol.

A number of other enzymes and molecules in the body are also important for dealing with toxins like heavy metals. They have a lot of crazy names: metallothioneins, divalent metal transporter 1, paraoxanase 1, glutathione, and methylenetetrahydrofolate reductase. Studies of mutations in the genes that code for these enzymes show they can have a profound effect on levels of heavy metals, such as mercury, lead, or cadmium, in your system, even if you work around them all of the time like car mechanics or other engineers do.

A less sophisticated way of exploring this involves your own personal and family history. Do you or anyone you know have a history of illness that can be traced back to toxic exposures? We are not talking about whether people have been exposed to toxins, but how well the body is able to respond to them. Ways of getting an answer to this question can start by looking at your family's history. Is there a preponderance of cancers or autoimmune disorders in your family? Do people in your family tend to get sick a lot?

Most important, how have *you* been throughout your life? If you have had chronic symptoms of any type, they could be related to your body's reaction to toxins. If you have been generally healthy, your body is obviously able to handle a great deal of toxic exposure since we are all living in a chemically toxic world. But before you get too comfortable, keep in mind that this is something all of us would be wise to be thinking about regardless of health status. You might be feeling good today, but your toxin burden could topple over tomorrow.

This leads us to the next, and perhaps most important, set of questions: "What types of toxins have you been exposed to, how much, and what exposures can you reduce starting now?"

The situation with an exploration of toxic burden is that it sometimes can be quite difficult, even impossible, to determine what types of toxins you may have been exposed to. But let's start from the beginning. Since you developed as a fetus in your mother's womb, do you have any evidence that your mother may have been exposed to various toxins? Did she smoke or drink alcohol? Did she have a lot of mercury fillings? Did she perform any jobs that may have exposed her to various chemicals, such as working with cleaning supplies, artist supplies, or as a metal worker? Did she ever live in an area known to have a high level of toxins such as on a farm, near a factory, or in certain cities? Did she mention that other people in your hometown had unusual diseases or cancers? And did she suffer any illnesses in her life, particularly around the time of her pregnancy with you?

The next important question is: "What toxins are you aware of having been exposed to?"

You can now ask some of these questions about yourself. Were you raised on a farm or in an area that had excessive toxins? Do you have a lot of mercury fillings in your mouth? Have you had any surgery in which some type of metal or molecular compound may have been placed into your body, such as orthopedic hardware or breast implants? And do you do any activities like work with machines, arts and crafts, or cleaning chemicals? Also, what types of foods have you eaten throughout your life? Have you eaten mostly organic natural foods or highly processed ones? Have you eaten meats that were produced with the use of antibiotics and hormones? Have you eaten fruit and vegetables that were grown with the use of pesticides?

If your answer is yes to any of these questions, the next step is to try as best as possible to determine what toxins you have been exposed to. If you worked with machines, it could be various chemicals that are involved with metals. If you lived on a farm, it could be numerous pesticides, antibiotics, or hormones.

A variety of tests for these are available, but they are often controversial.[3] Perhaps the most widely used test looks for heavy metals, usually in the blood. A blood test for these toxins is typically available at most laboratories. However, there are a number of other ways of testing for toxins in your body. They can be performed with a urine sample or sometimes a hair sample. Other times, the test can be performed with a chelating agent with the goal of trying to force excretion of the metal into the urine and then testing the urine. Such lab works are also called *provocation tests* to provoke the release of the metals. Most of these tests, however, are not currently approved by the Food and Drug Administration (FDA) and their accuracy and quality are often questionable.

But even if these tests were accurate, they show the presence of the toxin only in the serum or the urine. This does not necessarily imply that the toxin is or is not in the brain. Furthermore, if the toxin is in the brain, it is not clear how that relates to the amount of toxin in the rest of the body; the amount in the brain could be more, the same, or much less. However, the most important aspect of this thought process is for you to become more aware of the toxins in your environment and to implement changes that will give your system some room to heal and rebound from whatever has happened in the past. The deep exploration of past exposure is something we focus on with patients who are ill and have hit a wall in their conventional care. If that doesn't sound like you, then keep thinking about things to maximize your brain-body health.

Another approach to evaluating toxins is through a porphyrin test. Porphyrins are molecules that play a part in the production of hemoglobin in red blood cells. Some people have inborn errors of metabolism that create high levels of porphyrins called porphyria. It is a serious illness that can result in a variety of neurological and psychiatric symptoms. Most people do not have porphyria, yet the porphyrins may have an ability to indirectly indicate the presence and effect of various toxins. Toxins have been found to disrupt a number of enzymes involved in processing porphyrins. In a porphyrin diagnostic test, a urine sample is typically sent to a lab where specific porphyrin molecules are measured. If they are elevated, the implication is that a toxin involved in the processing of that porphyrin may be causing a backlog accumulation. The accumulation of specific porphyrins can then be tied to the presence of toxins such as mercury or various organic compounds. The downside of the porphyrin test is that it is often not too specific. It is not a direct measure of a specific toxin, and thus any abnormalities may not be clearly linked to the presence of a given toxin. However, it helps paint the picture of where physiology has been affected and offers a lab value we can track.

The goal of any of these investigations always is to maximize function and quality of life by restoring optimal brain-body health, so back to the good news: just because you come in contact with a toxin—and you assuredly will—does not mean that your body is going to have a problem with it. However, given what we know about toxins, you want to avoid a high toxin burden as much as you can in order to keep the tremendous resilience and detoxification systems in your body functioning at their best and to keep you in your healthiest possible state.

TOXINS TO BE CONCERNED ABOUT

Heavy Metals

Heavy metals are a common toxin that everyone has to be aware of. Certainly there are some obvious ones such as mercury and lead. Others that are also potentially problematic are cadmium, arsenic, and manganese.

One of the most common sources of mercury toxins are dental fillings. Mercury dental fillings were more common in the past, but some fillings continue to have small amounts of mercury. The other major source is from fish and seafood since there many waters have mercury in them. In terms of avoiding mercury exposure, one approach is to avoid dental fillings that have mercury in them, and another is to consume wild fish and seafood from cold waters such as near Alaska or similar northern areas.

It is controversial as to whether removing fillings that are already in place is a good idea.[4] Getting the mercury out of your mouth is beneficial, but some evidence suggests that the entire process of extracting the fillings ends up exposing you to more of the mercury leaching in through the bloodstream and the gut. If you just leave the fillings in, whatever mercury they have may no longer be entering your system.

In terms of mercury in your water, you can try to test for heavy metals and use bottled or filtered water that has had these metals removed. When it comes to seafood, certain types seem to be more problematic than others. Fish with the highest amount of mercury that are also common on dinner plates include swordfish, mackerel, tuna, cod, orange roughy, and American lobster. While fish have other health benefits for the brain such as good oils, they must be eaten in moderate amounts so that the mercury issue does not become a greater concern.

Lead is found in water as well, but the greatest exposure from lead appears to occur in household and building paints. Many children have been exposed to lead in their schools, especially in those that are fairly old. Other sources of lead can come from the air, soil, and water and frequently result from the burning of fossil fuels. However, most gasoline these days is unleaded. But lead can be found in many other sources, including pipes, faucets, food containers, and cigarette smoke. Since lead is everywhere, it is difficult to avoid completely. So take care to remove obvious sources such as lead paints or lead pipes in your home or workplace.

Lead is particularly problematic for brain development in children. Symptoms can include reduced intelligence and cognitive functioning, as well as emotional disorders. It may be difficult to completely fix the brain of someone who has been affected by lead, especially if the brain itself has already formed, usually by about age twenty-five. And lead may even lead to accelerated aging and brain deterioration as we age. However, there are some ways to help remove lead from your body and support your brain's function.

Cadmium, which has its origins in mining and smelting, is also relatively widely dispersed in the environment. It arises from the use of nickel-cadmium batteries and the production of various fertilizers, pigments, and plastics. There can be relatively high levels of cadmium in cigarette smoke because the tobacco plant takes up cadmium from the environment. Although cadmium does not cause a lot of direct neurological effects, it is believed to be a possible factor in a variety of neurodegenerative diseases including Parkinson's disease, Alzheimer's disease, and Huntington's disease. Cadmium also inhibits appropriate neuronal growth and development, and thus can be detrimental to children. As with all other heavy metals, there is only so much you can do to avoid exposure to it. Not smoking and trying to avoid areas of high pollution are typically the best ways of reducing your exposure.

Arsenic, another naturally occurring metal that may be a significant risk factor for cancers, can be found in contaminated drinking water, cigarettes, food, and various industrial production processes. Like other heavy metals, arsenic can harm the brain, mostly by causing dysfunction in the neurons, which can result in difficulties with cognition, memory, and mood. It may have a greater effect in younger individuals, particularly children who are still developing. However, adults can also suffer from neurological and psychiatric conditions associated with arsenic exposure.

Pesky Pesticides and Solvents

A variety of organic molecules can potentially be toxic to the human brain—for example:

- Solvents that cause damage to the nervous system, including n-hexane, perchloroethylene, and n-butyl mercaptan

- Solvents associated with liver or kidney damage, including toluene, carbon tetrachloride, (4) 1,1,2-2-tetrachloroethane, and chloroform

- Solvents known or thought to pose reproductive hazards, including 2-methoxyethanol, 2-ethoxyethanol, and methyl chloride

- Known or suspected solvent carcinogens, including carbon tetra-chloride, trichloroethylene, 1,1,2,2-tetrachloroethane, perchloro-ethylene, and methylene chloride

- Phthalates and bisphenol A, which can cause a variety of problems throughout the body

- Plastics, metals, and lubricants, which can cause a variety of prob-lems throughout the body

These organic molecules can also represent a variety of pesticides and fertilizers that become incorporated into the foods we eat and can cause a variety of problems at the neuronal level. Basic neuronal functions can be blocked, neurons cannot grow or form new connections as easily, and oxidative stress can result in the damage or destruction of neurons. Symptoms associated with exposure to organic molecules can include impairment to both cognitive and emotional processes.

GETTING THE LEAD OUT

If it has been clearly established that you have had some substantial exposure to heavy metals, and especially if you and your doctor believe it is causing symptoms, try to determine exactly which ones have been causing you to not feel well. As we have mentioned before, this is a complicated issue because many symptoms can be caused by a variety of metals and other toxins. Once the specific toxins are determined, you can use a variety of approaches t to get them out of your system, and out of your brain.

The body naturally helps to detoxify itself over time, so one of the most important things to do is to remove the environmental source of the toxin. Think about what it would be like to use a small bucket to bail out a boat with a large hole in its bottom. If you don't fix the hole and water keeps coming in, you will eventually sink. But if you can block the hole so that water no longer gets in, eventually you can keep the boat afloat. Similarly, if you can remove the ongoing exposure to the toxin, your body will naturally help to remove it over time.

In fact, one of the most important things is to watch the number of foods you eat that could potentially have toxins. Eating natural foods, organic foods, and foods that help eliminate toxins can be beneficial to reducing the overall burden they pose on your system.

Foods that can help eliminate toxins include cruciferous vegetables such as cauliflower, kale, and broccoli, and leafy greens, which have antioxidant and anti-inflammatory effects, as well as cleansing effects specifically from their chlorophyll.[5] Green tea has antioxidants and helps to stimulate the production of detoxification enzymes in the body. Beets and beet juice can also augment various detoxifying enzymes. Avocados have a lot of antioxidants, and their fatty acids have been shown to protect against damage caused by d-galactosamine, a powerful liver toxin. Cilantro can enhance mercury excretion and decrease lead absorption. Ginger and turmeric have strong antioxidant activity. Several fruits can be helpful too. For example, the pectin in apples may help facilitate the excretion of mercury and lead. Lemons can protect liver function and prevent oxidative (stress-related) damage. Blueberries are full of antioxidants and also have been shown to increase the activity of the body's natural killer cells, which are important immune cells for fighting infection and cancer.

It is also essential to stay well hydrated because many toxins are water soluble. The more you drink, the more these toxins are excreted in your urine and cleared from your system. Furthermore, staying well hydrated allows cells to function at their optimal level so that they can also help to clear the toxins from your system as well as function as effectively as possible even when toxins are present.

Sometimes the body's ability to remove a toxin is insufficient for the amount of exposure. When this happens, there are other approaches that can help. A simple and fun way to remove them can be through the use of a sauna. Saunas help to increase the body's temperature with the goal to of excreting various toxins and metals through the skin surface.[6] Toxins that are fat soluble can be excreted through the exocrine glands, while toxins that are water soluble can be excreted through the sweat glands. The typical approach is to use a sauna two to four times a week for about fifteen to forty-five minutes a session and for a period of about eight to twelve weeks, always done with the advice of a trained health care provider who can determine if it is safe for you to experience the high temperatures. It is important that when you get out, you immediately take a shower in order to wash off any of the toxins that remain on your skin surface. If you don't shower, much of the toxin will be absorbed back in through the skin. So by removing them through showering, particularly by using a luffa sponge, you can begin to remove the toxins from your system in a gentle manner.

Few studies clearly document how well saunas and sweating might work to remove toxins. It's likely the amount removed is probably fairly small. It would be ideal to test the amount of toxin you find in your system initially and then again at the end of a period of time using the saunas to get a better sense of how effective it is for you. Of course, the most important thing is whether you feel better symptomatically.

Many health spas and gyms have saunas. Some people purchase or rent one for a period of time for use in their home. In fact, infrared saunas, which are supposed to provide more heat inside your body—the temperature inside becomes higher than the sauna air temperature—have become popular, although it is not clear that they work any better than standard saunas.

Another approach to removing toxins such as heavy metals is through the use of various chelating agents that bind the toxins to facilitate their removal from the body. Some of these agents are taken orally, and others are given intravenously. A fascinating study performed at the behest of the National Institutes of Health (NIH) found that using the chelating agent EDTA (ethylene diamine tetra-acetic acid) substantially reduced all-cause mortality, cardiovascular death, reinfarction, and stroke in patients with diabetes and known cardiovascular disease.[7] This came as quite a surprise to the standard medical establishment, and researchers are in the process of doing the next set of trials. Other studies have demonstrated improvement in cognition and emotional well-being in patients exposed to various toxins when given appropriate chelating agents.[8]

Oral chelating agents can include DMSA (dimercaptosuccinic acid or succimer) and zeolite. DMSA can be given orally or intravenously. Orally, absorption can be affected by the overall health of the gut. About a quarter of the DMSA taken orally is excreted in urine; it increases urinary excretion of arsenic, cadmium, lead, methylmercury, and inorganic mercury. It has also been shown to remove lead and methylmercury from animals' brains and thus promote healing.[9] Zeolites are porous minerals that help bind and remove various toxins and heavy metals.[10] It is essential to discuss these approaches with your physician since chelating agents must be used carefully, and the data on their clinical effectiveness are limited. Nevertheless, they can be right for the right type of person and issue.

MOLD TOXINS

Mold toxins represent another challenge for the brain that might be far more widespread than currently recognized. Molds and fungi are ubiquitous in the world. Anyone who has lived in an old home, apartment, or office building has probably been exposed to some type of mold or fungus. And in areas that are more tropical, there can also be extensive amounts of molds or fungus due to the humidity and heat.

Many different types of mold and fungus can affect the human brain and body. Molds include species such as *Cladosporium, Penicillium, Aspergillus, Alternaria,* and *Trichoderma. Stachybotrys chartarum* is a mold that particularly produces mycotoxins, which are toxin molecules produced by molds or yeast. *Candida,* a yeast, is a type of fungus and the most common cause of fungal infections. It can also produce toxins that affect the body and cause various physical and mental symptoms.

People can have an infection with a mold or fungus, but most of the time, fungal infections are superficial, such as vaginal yeast infections or infections of the scalp and genital areas, which often can be treated with topical, over-the-counter medications. However, some fungal infections can become invasive; cryptococcal meningitis and mucormycosis, for example, can affect the brain directly. These usually occur in patients who have compromised immune systems.

When it comes to mold and fungus, the body can react beyond just an infection. People can have allergic reactions to the mold or fungus itself. If you suspect that you are exposed to mold or fungus in your home or workspace, it might be worth getting tested for allergies against these organisms.

Many of these organisms produce a variety of toxins. There are over three hundred known mycotoxins, with the most common ones being aflatoxins, ochratoxins, and trichothecenes. As toxins, they can become incorporated into a variety of cells in the body, including brain cells. Once inside, the toxins can disturb many cellular processes that can lead to dysfunction and disease.

You can also have allergic reactions to the toxins. Here, the two main approaches to treatment are to remove the exposure and eliminate it from your body. Removing it from the environment sometimes requires remediation of a home or building. Companies can be brought in to test for mold and fungi and then remove them using a number of cleaning techniques. This can be essential, especially if you are in an area that has a known problem with it. Sometimes this is referred to as the sick-building syndrome. It may be important to know if other people in your building have had similar symptoms. You might even ask if they have had unusual symptoms or frequent illnesses that don't seem to have a ready explanation.

Part of the struggle with understanding how mold and fungus affect the brain is the lack of approved testing methods available. *Candida*, perhaps the most common, does have several blood tests that can be easily obtained and report whether you have antibodies to it; if you do, this implies exposure. And a number of allergen tests can also be effective for determining if you have an allergy to mold or fungus. But just because you are allergic doesn't mean that you have an active exposure. Just like people who are allergic to cats, if the cat is not in the room, they feel totally fine. There are several controversial approaches that use urine to assess for the presence of certain mold toxins. As with diagnostic tests for other toxins, one of the primary concerns is that these studies measure only toxins that are in the urine and do not identify what toxins specifically may be in the brain or body. These studies are typically expensive, not covered by insurance, and are not currently approved by the Food and Drug Administration. This does not mean they are useless, but it does mean that it's best to regard them with caution. It would be ideal to get an initial measure of toxic burden, go through a therapeutic process, and then measure again to see if it has been removed.

As with metals and other toxins, mold toxins can also be removed from the body. One large case series of one hundred patients evaluated a number of approaches that included the use of saunas, antioxidants, and anti-inflammatories.[11] Patients were treated by avoiding the mold, using allergy treatments such as desensitization techniques, and engaging in regimens that included saunas, oxygen therapy, and nutrients. In this report, approximately 85 percent of all patients completely cleared their symptoms, 14 percent had partial improvement, and 1 percent remained unchanged.

SYNTHETIC HORMONES

Synthetic hormones are another important toxin to be aware of. Our environment today has a number of synthetic hormones most often used for raising animals, but they even enter the environment when used as drugs for humans. In the latter, sometimes these hormones are used for the treatment of post-menopausal women to help improve symptoms or prevent bone loss. Other synthetic hormones can be used by men to help improve their muscle strength or performance. These anabolic steroids have been highly controversial over the years and have often resulted in athletes being banned or stripped of awards. Lance Armstrong, for example, had his seven Tour de France medals taken away. However, anabolic steroids also have medical uses; they can help people with growth complications or with wasting syndromes such as in cancer or AIDS. And there is a large group of steroids that includes hydrocortisone, prednisone, and many others used for medical purposes.

While all of these synthetic hormones can have benefits, those pluses occur when they are used for specific purposes under proper medical guidance. The concern is that many people end up getting these synthetic hormones when they don't need or want them. One result is that they are excreted by the body and get into the water supply and ultimately the soil, plants, and animals. And if you inadvertently take in these hormones, especially over long periods of time, there can be a lot of health consequences. They can cause hormonally related conditions as well as cancers associated with hormones such as breast or prostate cancer. They can influence your immune system throughout your body and gut and even affect your brain function.

As with all of the other toxins discussed in this chapter, the best approach is to avoid getting them in your body in the first place. Eating hormone-free meats and organic foods can help, but sometimes it is difficult to avoid them. If you are worried that you have been exposed to synthetic hormones, the question is whether you can remove them and reduce their effects. When it comes to many synthetic hormones, especially medications, the good news is they typically have a short half-life in the body, so aggressive detoxification is not necessary.

The not-so-good news is that synthetic hormones called xenoestrogens, which are toxins, are found in things such as plastics, beauty products, and cleaning supplies. Like the other synthetic hormones, xenoestrogens mimic your body's natural hormones, in this case, estrogen. However, they are not easily removed from the body and must be detoxified and eliminated through the liver into the gut. But if the liver or the gut is not working well, it might be difficult to eliminate them.

In the end, weaving together optimal brain functions involves a combination of reducing your exposure to various toxins; watching your diet and nutrition, which helps reduce exposure and helps clear toxins you may already have; and using appropriate approaches for removing toxins when necessary. If you can do these things, you may be able to help keep your brain as healthy as possible for as long as possible.

Chapter 5

BRAIN GAMES: DO THEY WORK?

The brain has muscles for thinking as the legs have muscles for walking.
—JULIEN OFFORY DE LA METTRIE, 1747

When it comes to weaving yourself a great brain, the best way to think about this is by using the analogy of a muscle: the more you train the muscle and the more you use it, the better it typically functions. But there are lots of different ways of training muscles and brains for optimal functioning.

One of the most important distinctions is the difference between exercises that have a general effect versus those that have a specific effect. If you want to become a good tennis player, for example, you have to practice tennis as much as you can. Practicing something else—say basketball—will not help you much with your tennis game. In that sense, practicing tennis is a specific way of training your muscles. And the more you train, the more your muscles learn how to do all of the appropriate moves in order to hit the ball in the best way possible. Your leg muscles learn the appropriate footwork, your back muscles learn how to pivot into the ball for power, and your arm and hand muscles learn the most effective way of delivering just the right torque on the ball. All of those activities are specific to playing tennis as optimally as possible.

So where does general training come into play? Tennis players need a great deal of strength and stamina, so running or lifting weights can be helpful in making you as good a tennis player as possible. But running and lifting weights are also useful for almost every other athletic activity. If you want to be a top ice skater, cyclist, baseball player, or any other type of athlete, running and lifting weights is essential. In that regard, running and lifting weights are a general form of activity that have benefits regardless of what specifically you do with your muscles.

The brain is similar. There are types of training and exercises that are good no matter what you want to use your brain for and types of training that strengthen specific skills. Activities that help your brain concentrate or help reduce stress and anxiety can be useful for anyone's overall brain function. But if you want to become a great mathematician. it makes much more sense to do lots of mathematical problems than it does to do crossword puzzles. In fact, the data typically show that the more you do a specific activity with your brain, such as crossword puzzles, the better you become at that activity. Thus, if you want to be a great chess player, practice and play lots of chess even though that activity will not necessarily make you concentrate better in other areas of your life.

It is also important to find the right balance between an appropriate amount of training and overtraining. Stressing your body is actually the only way to make it grow and develop. That's how lifting weights works. The stress starts out modestly and is increased incrementally. The initially small amount of stress on the muscles strengthens them so they become a little stronger over time. When you add the next level of stress, you will build up your strength until you are ready for more. But if you try to lift too much too fast, you will injure your muscles. The brain can become overloaded too. And neuroplasticity also develops through slow, gradual challenges. So if you want to achieve a college-level mastery of mathematics but have never had a math class in your life, you start with basic addition and subtraction. Then you work your way up to algebra and maybe even calculus. The trick is to find the right balance between stressful challenges and the necessary rest and recovery that are part of the most appropriate training to ensure that your brain learns and grows as optimally as possible. Some things to watch out for as clues that you might be overchallenging your brain to the point of too much stress are strong emotional responses such as anxiety, depression, or a sense of burnout. If you feel this happening, you might need to take a break and slow the progression of training. Also, if your brain feels as if it is giving out, meaning that you feel overwhelmed and cannot do the training, it is also time to take a break.

With these points in mind, we can delve deeper into whether various brain games help your brain perform its best. We'll look at both general and specific approaches.

GENERAL BRAIN TRAINING

When it comes to general training of the brain, we have to think about broader cognitive and emotional processes. Concentration and attention, memory, brain stamina, management of stressful or competitive situations, and even optimal social interactions are all broad processes of the brain that can be trained.

Concentration and attention activities can be found in lots of different areas. In fact, even specific training programs can promote concentration and attention. And some activities, such as meditation, can improve concentration and attention regardless of what you may use these processes for. Hence, meditation is a key method for general brain training.

A variety of meditation programs fall under the category of concentrative practices. What this essentially means is that during practice, you concentrate on a particular object. The object can be specific and distinct. such as a candle or even something you imagine in abstract form, like a walk through a forest. The object can also be a word, sound, or series of sounds such as a mantra you repeat over and over. And sometimes the object can be as simple as your breath itself.

These practices come by different names. One of the most common practices that involves a mantra is transcendental meditation. By repeating the particular mantra given to you over and over in your mind and sometimes out loud, you develop the concentrative processes of your brain. Another mantra-based practice is Kirtan Kriya, which arises out of the Kundalini yoga tradition. This practice is performed by repeating, usually singing, the following sounds over and over: Saa Taa Naa Maa. You first repeat them out loud for two minutes, then in a whisper for two minutes, then in silence for four minutes, then in a whisper for two minutes, and finally out loud for two minutes. As you repeat these sounds, add a mudra sequence by gently touching each finger to your thumb starting with your index finger, and moving individually to the next finger until you reach your pinky. This is meant to be done simultaneously on both hands. Repeat the mudra for each round of sounds. The whole practice takes twelve minutes.

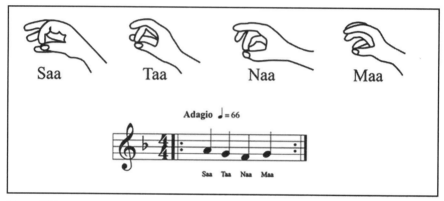

Kirtan Kriya practice.
ILLUSTRATION COURTESY OF THE ALZHEIMER'S RESEARCH AND PREVENTION FOUNDATION, COPYRIGHT 2003, 2015

When we studied this practice in older individuals, we found the Kirtan Kriya meditation increased activity by about 10 percent in the frontal lobe, the part of the brain that is particularly involved in concentration.[1] The participants also increased their ability to concentrate by about the same percentage. All of these changes occurred by doing this simple twelve-minute meditation practice once a day for eight weeks. So you can imagine how such a practice might help your brain improve concentration over a lifetime. Please see the brain imaging figures titled Meditation and the Brain in the color photography section for evidence of the benefits that meditation can offer.

Concentrating on your breath is the simplest practice of all. All you do is bring your focus to breathing in and out and trying not to think about anything other than your breath. If you notice yourself becoming distracted, don't get upset or frustrated; just immediately bring your attention back to your breath. As you do this over time, you will continue to increase your concentration powers. You can also incorporate this with a so-called body scan in which you bring your focus to each part of your body, starting with the top of your head and going down to your toes. Paying attention to each body part and any feelings it has, such as pain or discomfort, further supports your brain's ability to concentrate. In addition, the body scan can help you learn how your body is feeling, especially when it is stressed and when it is relaxed.

Awareness itself, which is related to concentration, is the basis of mindfulness or mindfulness-based stress reduction (MBSR), a meditation practice that we have studied in great depth. The goal of the mindfulness approach is to learn to be aware of the present moment, and nonjudgmentally. This awareness involves a type of concentration that allows for a space, so to speak, to navigate the stressors of life.

Interestingly, concentration has two basic processes. One of them is to positively or actively concentrate on a given action, task, or object. The other is to screen out interfering stimuli so that you can concentrate on the target. People who have attention-deficit hyperactivity disorder (ADHD) can have difficulty with either of these two processes or both at the same time. Some people have trouble concentrating on a particular thing, and some people are too easily distracted by other things.

Several studies have started to explore whether meditation practices might be useful for people with ADHD by helping them to improve their concentration. It seems that combining meditation practices with standard treatment can be useful in patients with ADHD. However, meditation by itself has not been shown to be effective. Of course, if the ADHD is too severe, medications may also be required in order to help the person even begin to concentrate during the meditation practice. The combination of both medication and meditation could potentially be valuable for those with this struggle.[2]

Religiously oriented practices such as contemplative prayer can have an effect similar to meditation if there is a concentrative element to them. A number of our own studies on spiritual practices that involve concentrating on a prayer or on God have shown that the frontal lobe becomes more active. The more you concentrate on a specific prayer or phrase from the Bible, the stronger you make your brain.

Interestingly, our earlier muscle analogy goes even further when considering how meditation practices affect the brain over the long term. A number of studies have shown that long-term meditators have thicker frontal lobes than those who are nonmeditators.[3] Since it is the frontal lobe that helps with concentration, meditation is like lifting weights for the brain. When you lift weights for a muscle, it becomes stronger and bigger. Similarly, when you lift "meditation weights" for the brain, it becomes stronger and literally bigger.

It is also possible that because a larger brain may help people avoid or stave off neurodegenerative disorders that result in the shrinking of brain size, a condition known as *brain atrophy*. Since Alzheimer's disease reduces the size of the brain, starting with a larger brain can help lessen the effects of the disease for a longer period of time. This cognitive reserve has been well documented in research. People with higher levels of education tend to have a better prognosis with diseases like Alzheimer's because their brain inherently is bigger in terms of volume and complexity. It has more reserve available to better withstand the Alzheimer's disease process that destroys brain cells. While the disease process itself may eventually overwhelm the reserves in place, those safeguards can have a significant protective effect. We discuss this more in chapter 18.

SPECIFIC BRAIN PRACTICES

There are thousands of specific types of practices that you can do for your brain, and doing any one of them primarily makes you better at that particular practice. Doing more crossword puzzles makes you better at doing crossword puzzles, and practicing the piano makes you better at playing the piano. These functions do not necessarily spill over into other ways in which the brain works. However, the more specific types of practices you do, the more broadly your brain will be able to function, which means that it seems reasonable to try to engage your brain in as many different ways as possible to keep it functioning as optimally as possible.

So you could do crossword puzzles on one day, play tennis on another, practice the piano on the next day, and watch a lecture on European history the day after that. By doing all of these activities, you help increase your brain's resilience and functionality.

While there are many common types of practices, neuropsychologists have developed a number of specific brain exercises that can be useful for supporting particular cognitive processes. In addition, a variety of computer training programs can help to develop your memory, language skills, concentration skills, or all of these. Research on the effect of these practices and activities has generally been quite positive. But if you need advanced training due to a brain injury or illness, working with a trained neuropsychologist is best. These medical professionals will first test you to gain a thorough understanding of your cognitive deficits and then select training programs and exercises tailored to your needs.

The data on the many online programs and apps that have been developed with the goal of helping people improve their brain function are somewhat lacking, but studies are increasing and more or less saying what we have all along: we might expect any specific activity to help you improve your abilities in that activity. With that in mind, programs such as Lumosity and BrainHQ have expanded their different types of activities so they can help with specific cognitive processes and perhaps the brain more generally.[4]

Studies in patients with strokes or head injuries show similar findings. One study of 115 stroke patients showed that an eight-week program on Lumosity resulted in some improvements more specifically related to the types of exercises engaged in, including working memory and processing speed. But in general, there were no more general improvements in cognitive functioning or quality of life.[5] Using the muscle analogy once again, if you were to pull your muscle, you might initially rest it, but then you would start to stretch and exercise it in order to bring its strength back to its original state. Once there, you would resume specific practices to develop the skills you need that muscle for. Similarly, if you have some injury to the brain, whether through a physical injury, exposure to a toxin, or a neurodegenerative disease, doing a varied number of both general and specific practices will be necessary to help bring back functions that you may have lost.

The good news here about the brain is that it is capable of creating new connections and even growing new neurons. This neuroplasticity has been well studied and documented in medical science literature. It occurs throughout one's lifetime, but it's typically more active in younger individuals. The bottom line is that at any stage of your life, you have the ability to modify your brain through specific practices.

Even playing video games can lead to improved brain function by improving hand-eye coordination, concentration skills, and the ability to adapt quickly to novel environments. In fact, several studies have compared video game playing as an active control group with programs such as Lumosity and have generally found that both activities improve brain function about the same.[6]

There are no data to show that one particular program or app is more effective than any other. Nevertheless, as with many other things regarding the brain, the most beneficial activity or practice is probably the one that you enjoy doing, is something that you can do frequently, and that engages your brain in one or more ways to improve its cognitive function, so try different programs, apps, and activities. The more you do, as long as you don't overstress yourself, the more you will enjoy a well-functioning and efficient brain.

Chapter 6

SLEEP BETTER, THINK BETTER

Sleep is the best meditation.

—The Dalai Lama, 1989

Sleep is essential for weaving together a healthy brain. In fact, a number of research studies have demonstrated the essential value of sleep for maintaining cognitive and emotional functioning. Sufficient restful sleep is restorative. Insufficient sleep is destructive, causing systemic inflammation and lower overall resilience. But what are the factors involved with having good sleep and maintaining that pattern? And what can you do if you find that your resting is not optimal? Integrative medicine approaches turn out to be incredibly helpful when it comes to improving sleep. The best sleep often requires a multifactorial approach that involves what is referred to as sleep hygiene: specific practices that might help to support sleep, natural foods and supplements for those who are having difficulty with sleep, and even medications when necessary.

WHAT IS NORMAL SLEEP?

Sleep is a curious thing. We all sleep; in fact, every animal sleeps, including insects. But why do we sleep? Through our research using brain scans, we have found that the brain is always on in terms of receiving blood flow and having neuronal metabolism and functioning. This means that in the middle of the night, your brain can appear just as active on a brain scan as it does during the day. So what is going on here? If the brain truly does not shut off, what exactly is happening during sleep, and why is it important?

It might surprise you to know that sleep is so critical that if you don't get enough of it, you will die. This does not refer to pulling an all-nighter during college or getting little sleep on a red-eye flight. But if you were purposely kept awake without any sleep at all, after about three days you would be virtually psychotic, and by six or seven days, you would likely be dead.[1] It is no surprise that sleep deprivation is sometimes used as a form of torture. Some studies suggest that sleep deprivation actually leads to significant oxidative stress in the brain and gut, which can lead to cell death and eventually the person's death.[2]

For the average person, normal sleep is typically seven to eight hours per night. Ideally, that means sleeping throughout the night with no more than one awakening. Sleep has well-defined phases—rapid eye movement (REM) and non-REM, the latter of which has stages with characteristic electrical patterns, as measured by an electroencephalogram (EEG). The types of electrical activity, or brain waves, during these non-REM stages are described as alpha, theta, and delta. We cycle through the phases and stages throughout the night.

Stage 1 sleep is typically referred to as drowsiness or pre-sleep. It is characterized by a combination of decreased alpha activity and an increase in theta waves, which are very slow brain waves. Stage 1 sleep lasts only about ten to fifteen minutes. During stage 2 sleep, people become less aware of their surroundings, their body temperature drops, and their breathing and heart rate become regular. This stage also produces rapid rhythmic brainwave activity called sleep spindles. People spend almost half of their total sleep time in this stage even though it lasts for only about twenty minutes at a time.

During stages 3 and 4, your deepest sleep occurs in delta waves, which are deep and slow brain waves. Your muscles relax, and your blood pressure and respiration decrease. Also during this stage, it is more difficult to wake up. Interestingly, sleepwalking occurs most often during stage 3 sleep. The most restorative sleep occurs during this time as well. It is when the body repairs and builds cells and tissues responsible for everything from muscle mass to immune function. As we age, we tend to get less non-REM sleep. People under thirty have about two hours of restorative sleep every night, whereas those over sixty-five have about thirty minutes. We'll discuss ways of maximizing this important stage of sleep.

The best-known stage of sleep is REM sleep in which the brain becomes more active even while the body becomes more relaxed and immobilized. It is called REM because our eyes move quickly and actively during this state. Importantly, it is during REM sleep that dreams occur. Research suggests that we spend about 20 percent of our total sleep time in this stage. The first period of REM typically lasts ten minutes, and the final period lasts about an hour.

When sleep is disrupted, one or more of these stages does not occur with the same amount or frequency, which can have far-reaching implications in terms of brain health and function. If everyone is deprived of sleep for approximately twenty-four hours, two groups of people tend to emerge: some function relatively normally, while others have significant impairments and dysfunction. But by seventy-two hours without sleep, everyone is a mess.[3]

More recent research has shown that even small reductions in overall sleep, especially over long periods of months or years, can lead to poor cognition, depression, and other emotional concerns. There is, of course, a bit of a vicious cycle that occurs. For those having difficulty sleeping because of emotional distress, poor sleep will compound their experience of uneasy emotions, thus making them less emotionally and physically resilient. In such situations, we first try to quickly find a natural solution, and if that does not work, we consider short-term medical interventions.

There is even evidence that poor sleep is associated with Alzheimer's disease and its resulting reductions in cognition. One of our clinical studies showed that poor sleep was associated with a greater accumulation of amyloid protein in the brain, a problematic protein that accumulates particularly in patients with Alzheimer's disease.[4] This is one of many studies in the recent literature demonstrating the pathological consequences of poor sleep.

Data even show that poor sleep can be every bit as bad as being drunk. Studies of people performing driving tests have shown that their significant reductions in sleep resulted in driving impairments that are similar to those who are intoxicated on alcohol. Their reaction times and perceptions of the environment fell, and they were much more likely to have an accident.

For these reasons, a number of industries and the military have been particularly interested in understanding sleep and the effects of sleep deprivation on the brain. People in transportation, the medical field, shift work, and the military have all experienced sleep-related problems and reduced brain function. So if your sleep cycles are messed up because you just did a couple of night shifts and were unable to sleep sufficiently during the day, or if you are a truck driver who just pulled an all-nighter to make a delivery on time, you need a period of restfulness before getting behind the wheel again.

The main reason these types of jobs are difficult has to do with the day-night cycle that our bodies are designed to follow. We have circadian rhythms that are regulated primarily by the day-night cycle or, more specifically, the light-dark cycle. It turns out that our body runs on a twenty-four-hour internal clock that is set by light and dark periods and regulated by neurotransmitters such as melatonin. That is why you will always feel most tired at night when it is dark, and even if you don't sleep much overnight, you will still start to feel more awake as the sun rises. Millions of years of evolution have set it so that we sleep at night to rejuvenate the brain and avoid being awake when night predators are about. So when your body is forced into a pattern that is different from the light-dark cycle, it does not work well.

One of the most interesting situations involving sleeplessness is with astronauts. Spacecraft often orbit the earth fifteen to twenty times per day. That means fifteen to twenty sunrises and sunsets in a twenty-four-hour period—more specifically, fifteen to twenty periods of light and dark. It is no wonder that astronauts suffer from a large number of sleep-related issues, and if they are not sleeping well, they may not perform or think well. When you are 150 miles up in space with nothing but vacuum around you, you cannot afford to make a mistake, so NASA and other spaceflight programs around the world have paid a lot of attention to making sure that astronauts sleep sufficiently by using a variety of the types of interventions we describe below.

Finally, it is important to note that some people sleep excessively. This is sometimes an indication of an underlying issue such as narcolepsy, sleep apnea, depression, or a variety of neurological and medical concerns including neurodegenerative diseases or cancer. These disorders can disrupt sleep patterns or cause excessive amounts of fatigue. While most people struggle with too little sleep, excess sleep isn't healthful either.

YOUR OWN SLEEP PROGRAM

In order to help you achieve your optimal sleep to make sure you have a healthy brain, let's start with thinking about you as an individual: Is sleep a strength or weakness of yours? Several basic questions can help you answer this:

Do you feel that you slept well last night?
Do you wake up more than two times most nights?
Do you sleep seven to eight hours most nights?
When you wake up in the morning, do you feel rested and full of energy?

These questions are just a start, but if you think that your sleep is typically impaired, we need to delve a bit deeper into the cause.

CAUSES OF POOR SLEEP

The most common cause of sleeplessness is related to external stressors. Virtually everyone has felt that they don't sleep well when they are under a lot of stress, whether that stress comes from a job, relationship, or health issue. It has to do with what's called the *autonomic nervous system*. This system has two sides: an arousal side, called *sympathetic* and commonly referred to as "fight or flight," and a quiescent side, called *parasympathetic* and commonly referred to as "restoration and recuperation."

During a regular day, it is normal for the arousal side to be on a bit so that you feel motivated to do all the activities that you need to do for optimal survival. And when you are under added stress, the arousal system kicks in even more. Another way of looking at this is that things that cause you stress are those that you perceive on some level to be a threat to your well-being. Hence, the fight-or-flight mechanism lights up, while the calming or quiescent side turns on when it is time to relax and rejuvenate your energy stores. The quiescent side is also the part of the autonomic nervous system that turns on when you're getting ready for sleep. Under most circumstances, the arousing and the calming sides of the autonomic nervous system usually inhibit each other. This means that when the arousal system kicks in, it suppresses the calming system, and vice versa. Of course, this makes sense since you would not want to feel that you need a nap when you are about to go into an important meeting. But the opposite is exactly what happens when you have a lot of stressors in your life and are trying to fall asleep. The calming system normally shuts your arousal system down unless it is on overdrive from too many underlying stressors. If your nervous system is registering that you are unsafe, perhaps even threats to your safety, the arousal system stays on, making it difficult to fall asleep. Thus, these external stressors, as well as the internal ones that our brain adds on top, such as our own anxieties, worries, and negative thinking, can make for a lot of tossing and turning.

Many of our stressors are not as big a threat when we create some space between us and them. That is what meditation and even prayer often allow us to do. We address these techniques and others in upcoming chapters. In addition, sometimes just taking an objective inventory of your stressors is helpful because the logical part of your brain and the emotional part of it that register stress often don't communicate, so an objective appraisal of how threatening the stressor really is can help put things in perspective. Think about all of the situations, people, and events that are causing stress in your life, and write them down in a list. Maybe you listed items like a new baby, a frightening pandemic, a sick parent, a major deadline at work, and financial worries. Rate each one of them on a scale of 0 to 10, with 10 being the most stressful thing you could ever imagine. Then ask yourself the following question about each one: "What am I saying to myself about myself in regard to this stressor?" Write down your answer and don't be surprised if it is illogical, such as "I'm trapped," even though you know that you aren't. Or you might be saying something that is an accurate appraisal of the situation. But you won't know until you ask. Finally ask yourself, "What emotions am I feeling such as fear, anger or sadness in regard to each of the stressors?" Now, when you have difficulty falling asleep, try to reflect on the statements you are saying to yourself and the emotions you are feeling. This will allow you to be more in touch with the effects particular stressors are having on your ability to enjoy restful sleep. This exercise will also prepare you to incorporate techniques like mindfulness and Neuro Emotional Technique (NET), which we discuss in greater detail in chapter 10.

Another common cause of sleeplessness has to do with your sleep hygiene: other behaviors that affect sleep. Do you watch television in bed when you ought to be asleep? Do you look at your smartphone or computer screen right before going to bed? That excessive light stimulation can make it difficult to get good rest. If you live in a city where a lot of sirens and other noises punctuate the night, that can also make it difficult for you to maintain your sleep level. Eating or exercising too close to going to bed can make it difficult to fall asleep too. It's also important to go to bed at approximately the same time every night. So if you aren't getting the kind of quality sleep you would like, take stock of how you prepare yourself for sleep and the environment in which you are sleeping. Are your bed and pillow comfortable? Can you eliminate noise or use a white-noise machine to drown out stimulating sounds and help you sleep? Can you do activities before going to bed that help you relax, such as reading or listening to calming music, rather than watching television or using the computer or smartphone? A lot of research has shown that simply improving your sleep hygiene can result in better sleep.[5] And interestingly, cognitive behavioral therapy can be effective for people with insomnia since it helps them work through the psychological causes of their sleeplessness.[6] In general, cognitive behavioral therapy is designed to help people modify their unhelpful thoughts, improve emotional regulation, and develop useful coping strategies targeting specific issues or behaviors.

Sleep apnea, a medical condition in which a person momentarily stops breathing in the middle of his or her sleep cycles, is another common cause of sleeplessness. When people with apnea stop breathing, their arousal system kicks in to say that it's time to take a breath and so it wakes them up. Sleep apnea is most common in people who are overweight because the added tissue will constrict around their windpipe when they lie down. However, about a quarter to a third of patients with sleep apnea are not overweight. For these individuals, the apnea is a result of other conditions such as enlarged tonsils, anatomical abnormalities that block airflow, endocrine disorders, acid reflux, lung disease, or heart disease. Frequently those with sleep apnea are heavy snorers. Often the condition is first noticed by the person they are sleeping with because the momentary pause in breathing followed by a gasp for air wakes them up as well. If this sounds like you, the best step is to talk to your doctor about getting a sleep study. These are done at a hospital, a hotel, or your home. Essentially the study measures your respirations as well as your oxygenation levels while you sleep. If the test shows that you stop breathing a number of times during the night and your oxygen levels fall, you may be diagnosed with sleep apnea.

There are a number of treatments for sleep apnea. If it is mild, sometimes treatments for other sleep issues like bruxism (teeth grinding) and loud snoring can help, such as a bite plate your dentist can make, over-the-counter nasal strips, or a nasal dilator. For more difficult cases, your doctor can prescribe an oral device to be fitted. The best-known mechanical device for this condition is a continuous positive airway pressure machine (CPAP), which can help keep the airway open throughout the night. It can work effectively, but its main downside is that it can also be uncomfortable or disturbing to wear and use.[7] There are also more aggressive options if all else fails, such as surgery.

Another cause of sleep issues can be from various medical concerns and their treatments. For example, any medical condition associated with pain or altered sensory stimuli in the body can interfere with sleep. Patients with chronic pain, including those with cancer pain, musculoskeletal conditions, fibromyalgia, and irritable bowel syndrome, can find sleeping difficult. Even medical conditions that do not have pain can sometimes have this effect on sleep. Patients with diabetes, high blood pressure, heart disease, and other serious issues all report reductions in their sleep. This can create a vicious circle since sleep is an important component of the healing process.

Beyond the medical conditions themselves, their treatments, including a wide variety of prescription medications, can interfere with appropriate sleep. The most common ones that interfere are those that directly affect the brain, such as some antidepressants and stimulants used to treat attentional disorders. And there are plenty of over-the-counter ones that can have a big negative effect on your sleep, such as drugs with pseudoephedrine for allergies and colds, headache medications that are loaded with caffeine, and energy products that often have stimulants in them. If you believe that you are not sleeping well, it is important to review with your doctor all of the medications and supplements you're taking. For some medications that have a stimulating effect, you might be able to change the timing of when you take them, or your doctor may be able to suggest alternatives that have fewer side effects.

WEAVING TOGETHER A MORE RESTED BRAIN

As you address and reconcile how to get restful sleep, you will manifest a healthier brain. When you improve your sleep and optimize your normal sleep structure—meaning the appropriate amount of each of the sleep stages, you will also improve your brain's overall function.

Stress

Let's start with the first issue that we just discussed: stress. Addressing stress requires a proactiveness on your part that might be different from what you are used to. However, the potential benefits of doing so are enormous. It is important to know how much stress you're under and whether that stress is truly affecting your sleep. Many of us walk around knowing we have big stressors but at the same time are disconnected from the internal effects they are having on us. The bad news is that unchecked stress can significantly impair your overall sleep quality. The good news is that there are proven ways of navigating stress so it doesn't get the best of you. In chapter 10, we discuss some effective stress reduction techniques that can be useful in general and also those specifically for around bedtime that can help soothe your stress as part of your sleep routine. Stress reduction programs and relaxation exercises can reduce the amount of stress that you have, reduce the activity in your arousal system, and allow your calming system to kick in as best as possible. In fact, a growing number of studies have shown that mindfulness-based programs and other meditation-based programs help to improve sleep duration and sleep quality.[8]

Of course, the best way to reduce stress is to find ways to help stop it altogether. This may not always be possible, but sometimes just taking a break such as a vacation or retreat, or even being more assertive in making important life decisions about work, relationships, and so on, can give relief.

Sleep Hygiene

The next important approach for improving your sleep is to improve your behaviors around it. This is particularly important for developing your own optimal sleep program. Consistency is the key to success, and again, this requires some proactive changes. At least two hours before going to bed, begin the process of winding down. Stop watching television, especially the news or anything else that will activate your brain, and turn off your computer. Read a little or connect with your partner or catch up with someone you care about on the phone. Create a ritual for washing up, getting ready for bed, or doing a relaxation exercise as we describe later. Maybe even light a candle for a few minutes that has a relaxing aroma such as lavender or lemon verbena, or whatever else feels soothing to you. These regular practices can help you find your most restful night's sleep.

In terms of biorhythms, we believe the ideal time to be asleep is by 10:00 p.m., or earlier if you like. One hour before your bedtime, which is best if it's at the same time every night, retreat to your bedroom. Look at the area where you sleep. Are there things you can do to make it more of a nighttime sanctuary? Are there bright lights you can turn off or block out? Can you use a white noise machine so that you don't hear disruptive noises? Make your sleep area neat and a place you want to be. If you have a partner, engage that person in the process.

Make sure that your mattress is s comfortable, and consider getting a new one if it is not. When you shop for a mattress, try different ones that give different degrees of support. Some are built for people who like to sleep on their side versus their back versus their stomach. You might even look at ones that are adjustable for firmness or positioning of the body. Also try different pillows. You may think that a soft pillow is what's best for you, but you might also discover that a firm pillow ends up helping you sleep more soundly. Or it might be the other way around. You won't know until you try several options.

Exercise

We all feel tired when we exercise a lot, so it is no surprise that studies find that a regular exercise program is essential for good sleep. It is always good to move around throughout the day, and the more you exercise, the more tired you will be at night and the better you will sleep.[9] Aerobic exercise at moderate intensity about three to five days per week has generally been shown to be effective for improving sleep quality and duration of sleep. However, be careful to leave at least three to four hours between your exercise and going to sleep or else the exercise can energize you and keep you up.

Sleep Aids

Many people find that sleep aid interventions are helpful. One of them takes advantage of something you are already familiar with. Almost all of us have fallen asleep in the back of a car or on a train because of the vibrations and sounds that the moving vehicle makes. As it turns out, research is demonstrating that specific rhythms associated with the vibration and sound stimuli can help lull the brain into the right rhythm for sleeping.

We studied one system that combined vibratory and auditory stimulation as part of a program to help people sleep better.[10] We took thirty-nine people with insomnia and randomized them to receive the stimulation or to be in the control group. The vibratory and auditory stimulation had two components. The vibratory system used a special bed that vibrated at frequencies with a goal of helping the brain get into the right sleep rhythms. People used this bed twice a week. In addition, they were given an audio program that played sounds of similar rhythms, again with a goal of getting the brain into the right sleep rhythms. Participants played this auditory stimulation program for about forty-five minutes each night before going to bed. The subjects did all of this for one month. We had scanned their brains before and after the program, and what we found was quite remarkable.

It turns out that the vibratory and auditory stimulation program affected several specific areas of the brain, some of them involved in receiving vibratory and auditory stimulation. Thus, the body perception centers and the hearing centers were substantially changed as a result of going through this program. This made sense and helped to confirm that the vibratory and auditory stimuli had an impact on the brain. We also observed changes in other areas of the brain that are affected by sleep deprivation and are associated with various cognitive and emotional processes. This study suggested that various programs that use vibrations and sounds can potentially be effective at helping people sleep better. You might want to try some type of similar program through your physician or by going online. The brain imaging figures titled Vibro-Auditory Therapy for Insomnia in the color photography section demonstrate the effectiveness of this program. You can also learn more about the studies and program we use in our clinic by going to marcusinstitute.jeffersonhealth.org.

A number of dietary supplements may support healthy sleep, though most have limited empirical data to back them up. Some of these are well known.

Melatonin is one that is fairly well researched and has a plausible scientific rationale to support it. Melatonin is a natural molecule that your body produces in response to the normal circadian rhythms, which control your light-dark cycle. As we age, many of us produce lower amounts of this molecule, which can affect sleep. Melatonin can also become dysregulated when traveling across time zones or under conditions of stress. We often consider recommending melatonin for people who are still having difficulty falling and staying asleep even after they have implemented good sleep hygiene. Dosage recommendations vary due to the different types of studies that have been done, but many people respond well to 3 to 5 milligrams about an hour before bedtime. This can be particularly effective when traveling and the normal light-dark cycle is physically altered because of time zone changes. Melatonin is generally safe at these doses and can be taken for long periods of time. Some people are sensitive to this supplement and feel groggy at the suggested dosage, so we often recommend they start with a small test for a couple of days, such as 1 to 2 milligrams. Other folks need a little more than 5 milligrams to see an effect. So if you decide to try it, start slow but stay with it long enough to get the amount high enough. We generally recommend an upper limit of 8 milligrams a day.

Glycine and tryptophan are two amino acids available as supplements that may have natural sleep-promoting qualities. Both are found in various foods, including turkey, which is why you often feel sleepy after Thanksgiving dinner. Capsules or packets of these amino acids are mildly sedating so they can be effective in people with uncomplicated sleep issues. Both likely work by increasing serotonin levels, which are important for maintaining mood and sleep patterns. These natural compounds have few side effects, but certainly if you experience a symptom that might be associated with a supplement, stop it and see if the symptoms improve. You can then discuss with your doctor whether to consider restarting it.

Chamomile, another natural compound that can promote sleep, has a relaxing effect on the body and can help bring the brain into a more natural sleep mode. Drinking some chamomile tea or taking approximately 200 milligrams of chamomile about a half-hour before bed has been shown to improve sleep quality in some people. Besides, a relaxing, warm, caffeine-free tea is a nice addition to daily sleep hygiene in general.

Medications

Some medications can also be useful for promoting sleep. They must be taken with care because many of these sleep-promoting medications can alter the normal sleep architecture, meaning they can alter the right amount of each of the stages of sleep. But if you are having an acute problem with sleep—for example, in response to a major life event—it may be a good idea to discuss with your doctor whether it is reasonable to try some sleep medications. The most common over-the-counter products are antihistamines, such as Benadryl and Unisom, which can help you fall asleep, but often the sleep quality is not very good and can result in sleepwalking or other sleep disturbances.

Many of the prescription drugs widely advertised, such as Lunesta, Belsomra, and Ambien, have the potential to be effective in the right circumstances, but great care must be taken when using them. And it is important to try to limit the duration for taking them as you work toward creating and switching to an optimal sleep program for yourself. Otherwise, it can become difficult to stop them. If you are really struggling to sleep while trying the various integrative interventions we have described, talk to your doctor, or even a sleep expert, to help you get more fully evaluated for medical conditions that might be the underlying cause. And when necessary, they can appropriately guide you to the right medical intervention.

Alcohol

Some people have the misconception that drinking alcohol at night helps with sleep. However, the research is clear: while alcohol might in some cases facilitate falling asleep, the quality of sleep is poor. Alcohol inhibits the important, restorative deep sleep that we need.

AN INTEGRATIVE APPROACH TO SLEEP

In the end, we hope you will take seriously the importance of your sleep. It is essential for optimal brain health, enabling it to function as best as possible and helping it to ward off a variety of neurological and psychological concerns. Start today to create your own individualized program using the approaches we described that focus on good sleep hygiene, which can also include meditation or other spiritual practices, vibratory or sound interventions or both, and appropriate supplements. And when necessary, consider medical interventions and more formal evaluations. By applying an integrative approach, you can achieve your optimal sleep, which is part of your achieving overall optimal health and well-being.

Chapter 7
THE SOCIAL BRAIN

*The hardest thing for not only an artist but for
anybody to do is look themselves in the mirror and acknowledge,
you know, their own flaws and fears and imperfections and put
them out there in the open for people to relate to it.*

——KENDRICK LAMAR, 2015

The human brain is a social brain. That means we are hard-wired to connect with one another. From an evolutionary standpoint, there is survival value in this: being part of a herd puts most mammals in a better position than being alone. Even our health and sense of well-being are dependent on socializing. Numerous studies have confirmed that we are designed for social connectedness and that loneliness is linked to negative health outcomes and even shorter life spans. So in order to have your best brain, avoid isolation and stay connected to others. Of course, there may be the occasional person in your life for whom the interactions are so stressful it is best they are avoided when possible. But overall, go out of your way to ensure daily interactions with others, such as family, friends, colleagues, neighbors, a friendly store clerk, and everyone else. Let's take a deeper dive into the mechanisms of the social brain and how to use them for your best overall brain health.

Being social is a complex process that encompasses your thoughts, feelings, and behaviors. Beyond that, your words, intonations, facial expressions, and body language all contribute to social interactions. And what is particularly amazing about the brain is that it mirrors what other people are doing around us. We have what are called mirror neurons that literally mimic what others are doing. If we are around people who are happy, we are more likely to feel happy inside, whereas if we are around people who are angry, we are more likely to become angry. Here, an important caveat is warranted. People almost always prefer to listen to those with similar belief systems because that supports their own way of thinking. When the content resonates, this further strengthen the emotional connection with the other person. When the emotion is a hostile one, though, it may contribute to overall strife, contentiousness, and exclusion of others—too common in today's divided world.

Hence, there is a delicate balance for optimal brain health that for most people takes a bit of training and conscious effort. On the one hand, it is beneficial to have plenty of interactions where you resonate with someone else through both the logical and emotional parts of your brain and, on the other hand, to step back from negative emotional impulses when you don't agree with a person's viewpoint and still find a way to enjoy the connection and honor the person nonetheless. That is the key to a brain and body that thrives.

ANATOMY OF THE SOCIAL BRAIN

Given the tremendous importance of socialization, the brain has developed specialized parts that help us with social interactions. For example, the parietal lobe of the brain has a special structure, the precuneus, which is involved in helping us to feel sociable. This area of the brain helps us infer what other people are thinking and feeling. For example, when people are engaged in an intimate conversation in which there is a smooth flow of interactions between them, the precuneus becomes particularly active. It can even become active in you before the other person utters another word, and vice versa. In this way, your brain becomes so attuned to the other person's brain that it experiences what is called *neuronal resonance*: the two brains become highly interactive with each other via the precuneus, along with the prefrontal cortex, which helps us pay attention to one another.

When the precuneus works with another structure, the insula, which sits between the emotional centers of the brain and the higher-thinking cortex, we are able to empathize and understand others' emotions. In this way, we can understand when someone is happy and when someone is sad. This provides an important way to help us interact with others. Thus, we instinctively know to laugh with someone who is happy and to comfort someone who is sad. Brain scan research also shows that the precuneus and the prefrontal cortex are particularly involved with helping us assess the trustworthiness of a person by reading his or her face.

Another part of the brain, the fusiform gyrus in the temporal lobe, is highly involved in our ability to understand facial expressions. This face recognition area is essential for us to be able to interact effectively with others. We use this area of the brain to observe the lift in someone's eyebrows, the upturned lips, and the wide eyes of someone who is happy. We can distinguish that face from someone with a furrowed brow, pursed lips, and squinted eyes who is angry. That is why we can understand the nuance when someone says to us, "You're crazy!" as to whether he or she is angry or otherwise upset about something we've done or mean it in a joking, complementary way because this person finds something we've done to be funny. So if the other person says it with a smile, we recognize a positive meaning. The fusiform gyrus is highly sensitive to the many facial expressions we can make and thus helps us understand what those around us are thinking and feeling.

In addition, our own facial expressions are being evaluated by others all the time. People can know if you're happy or sad simply by looking at you, without either of you necessarily having to say anything. Similarly, our body language expresses a great deal about how we are feeling. If you relax your shoulders and arms, others know that you are friendly. If you've folded your arms and are frowning, they know that you are upset.

Original groundbreaking work by Paul Ekman, named by the American Psychological Association as one of the most influential psychologists of the twentieth century, and many others that followed revealed a universality to facial expressions in relation to specific emotions.[1] That is, they are part of our neurological hardwiring. Experiments show that people of different cultures can both exhibit and detect the emotions of a wide range of facial expressions even in those from cultures and languages different from their own. Smiling when happy, frowning when sad, furrowing eyebrows when angry, cringing when disgusted, and so on are human phenomena that unite all of us.

Importantly, some learning and training can manipulate this neurological system. Just as a feeling of happiness can elicit your smile, making an effort to smile regularly can help facilitate your own happier emotional state. Going out of your way to emanate and express the joy you can muster within yourself not only nurtures a more joyful and brain-healthy state for you; it also does the same for those you live with, work with, and encounter on the street. As we take this back to socialization, it is clear that you can create a positive feedback loop that feeds your brain with high-quality and fulfilling connections. That means it is worth paying attention to the kinds of facial expressions you typically make. Does your face typically appear to be happy, sad, angry? When you start paying attention by checking the mirror, selfies, videos, or asking trusted friends, you might be surprised to see that you've slipped into a pattern that does not add up to an optimal brain or an optimal life.

Some interesting research found that a gentle smile with soft eyes tends to be the kind of face people feel is most compassionate and most trustworthy.[2] We have sometimes referred to this as the Mona Lisa smile, which may help to explain why the painting is widely recognized as one of the greatest pieces of art in history. Though the subject and artistic quality in and of itself may not be particularly exceptional, many have commented that Mona Lisa's facial expression is what pulls everyone in. It is difficult to look away from those soft eyes that seem to follow us and the gentle smile that seems to make us feel pleasant. Recall the mirror neurons we discussed earlier that cause a reciprocal response to what you see around you. Consider surrounding yourself with things and people that will engender this Mona Lisa effect, and think about ways you can be a Mona Lisa for yourself and others.

You can start by practicing making that facial expression yourself. Look at your face in a mirror, and try to soften your eyes. Now allow a gentle smile to come. Be careful about showing your teeth; focus just on your lips and the smile itself. When we start paying attention to this expression, we realize how often we intuitively do it in our own daily lives. Having a mind-set of wanting to put people at ease so we can be the best healers for them facilitates this kind of facial expression. Remember that there is a bidirectionality to these things. Knowing this helps us to be especially mindful of our eye contact, facial expressions, and even body posture when someone else is particularly distressed and needs our help. Also keep in mind that research has shown that simply making good eye contact will help you with your social interactions in part by acknowledging that you are interested in what the other person is saying.

If you feel you have not been effective at social interactions, the good news is that you can learn and practice the things that don't come naturally to you. The biological value for you is worth the effort. You can also practice the body language part of it. Actors, for example, practice how their body moves and how they can use it to express an idea or emotion. Similarly, you can practice by trying to stand more openly, with your arms relaxed at your sides or bent slightly forward rather than folded, and you can gently relax your shoulders as well. All of these types of body movements can help others see you as calm and inviting as opposed to unpleasant or closed off from engaging.

Beyond practicing your own body and facial expressions, it is important to practice observing others. You can do this in any place at any time—maybe at a store, on a bus or subway, or just walking down the street. What do people's faces tell you about them? Can you infer whether they seem happy or upset? And then try to apply this people reading to those who are more immediately in your life. Can you listen more intently and observe more closely your family and friends when they are talking to you? Can you become more mindful of what they are trying to say and how they are trying to express themselves to you? Do they seem calm and happy or seem upset and sad?

In addition to focusing on their facial expressions and body language, listening deeply to their words is essential. When engaging someone in a conversation, take several deep breaths so that you can remain calm and focus your attention on everything they are saying. Then allow yourself to listen to exactly what they are saying rather than simply reacting. Allow them to express themselves freely. Ask them brief and sensitive pointed questions. Our research shows that the more we engage in communication with others using this compassionate stance, the more compassion we feel toward others.

One of our colleagues has notoriously observed that medical students lose their compassion as they go through medical school.[3] This is likely because they spend a significant period of time in the medical education system with a disconnect between the science of the human body and the human being who is the patient. In response to this unfortunate situation, our medical school at Thomas Jefferson University, the Sidney Kimmel Medical College, has taken a leading role in educational reform and completely revamped its curriculum, focusing on case-based learning, bedside manner, and the patient experience. Another tremendous historical step is our medical school's creation of the first-ever full clinical department of integrative medicine, which is increasingly contributing to the curriculum of compassionate, patient-focused communication and care.

What we find from teaching and practicing this way, which you will also discover for yourself as you become more mindful of these approaches in your own life, is that you become more compassionate and understanding with others as well as with yourself. This is fundamental to having an ideal brain. If you can listen to your own thoughts and feelings more attentively and more deeply, you will have a better understanding of what you are experiencing and expressing. The more you are in touch with your own thoughts and feelings, the better able you will be to create positive connections with others and a greater sense of personal well-being.

CREATING SOCIAL NETWORKS

An expansive body of research shows that people with the most robust social network systems typically live the longest and cope with various problems in life the most effectively. In the medical world, patients fighting a number of diseases, including deadly cancers, will find greater quality of life if they have strong social networks. In fact, the research shows that people with the greatest support can live up to twice as long as those who do not.[4] For example, on a practical level, when we are faced with health challenges, social networks can provide us help with keeping appointments, taking medications, staying engaged in life activities, and helping out generally. They also profoundly help to ease anxiety and depression. Hence, creating strong social connections can make the good times more pleasurable and filled with more positive emotion and diminish the stressfulness of challenging times.

We have underscored the importance of your social network, but who comprises that network and how you balance your time across it depends on the circumstances. For example, you might have a large family, but the dynamics are mostly contentious, with a lot of anger. In that case, you might want to select the family member or two with whom you have a good connection and foster those relationships while minimizing engaging in the negative dynamics of the others. Or you might have a close nuclear family, and it makes sense to add some people from outside to broaden your social experiences. You might be single and living in a city far from your family of origin, in which case it might make sense to explore community opportunities to connect with others and create friendships. It is ideal to have some people you are extremely close to and whom you can rely on for help with many life issues. But the brain also likes to have many acquaintances and friends who might share specific interests such as sports, art, music, or video games. As we discussed in chapter 5, the more different ways you engage your brain, the better it works. Similarly, the more different types of people you can include in your social network, the better your brain functions. But again, it is always ideal to have a few people you can truly rely on in a deep and meaningful way.

David Brooks, a well-known political commentator, wrote in his book *The Social Animal* that as we go through our educational system, we are taught how to do mathematics or about who won World War II, but rarely are we taught how to engage socially with others.[5] It seems that we are just expected to know how to do it. But creating, establishing, and maintaining good relationships is not always easy. Anyone who has been in an intimate relationship for more than a few years knows that it often takes a great deal of work and regular compromise. It is necessary to never take for granted that we understand what the other person is thinking and that deep listening and paying attention to body language and facial expressions are essentials.

We have also performed research to learn how open-minded people are toward those who hold other beliefs or have a different ethnicity from our own.[6] It turns out it is likely that you, as is true for many of us, have a moderate amount of openness, but it is also important to always challenge your beliefs and biases that might prevent you from positively engaging with those from different backgrounds.[7] Based on how we understand the brain, it seems reasonable that the more you engage with people from all kinds of backgrounds, the more your brain will be stimulated and the better it will work. The only caveat is that the interactions be positive rather than negative. Getting into fights and increasing feelings of anger or hatred are detrimental to your brain.

While some people just naturally make more friends than others, there is a lot you can do to optimize the way in which your brain operates socially. And research shows that the social brain is something that can learn and develop. We have already mentioned some approaches. Though we all have to find our own path to creating a social network that is as effective as possible, it is always a good idea to keep exploring new relationships to challenge your brain and to have your social network system adaptable enough to withstand losing even close relationships.

PETS AND THE BRAIN

A discussion of how our brain interacts with others wouldn't be complete without exploring the human relationship with our furry and feathered and sometimes scaly friends. In today's world, many people turn to pets as a way of helping them to feel better, feel loved, and have fun. Few other experiences in the world can bring as much joy and pleasure to our lives. And while pets are not for everyone, if you like animals, owning a pet can be a wonderful source of support for your brain's functions.

Pets give us so much, but they also need us for their own survival. Their reliance on us teaches compassion and understanding and instills in us a sense of meaning and purpose. We also learn from our animal friends about the nature of life. I've always been so impressed that a dog chases a ball with unbounded enthusiasm even though he makes no money and gains no fame from actually getting that ball. It is just the pure joy of the chase. That basic element of life can be a great teacher about the relative importance of so many things that we think are important. Sometimes just the simple joys in life—cuddling, running, playing— are what we need to focus on in order to provide us with the greatest sense of overall well-being that is also good for our brain health.

Enjoying pets and animals has gone one step further through pet therapy. You may have seen various animals being guided through a hospital or airport in order to interact with people as a way to help them feel more comfortable and at ease. Pet therapy has been validated by an increasing number of research studies as a way to help reduce anxiety and depression for patients with various conditions, as well as for those in generally good health.[8] Of course, having a pet always needs to be balanced with other aspects of life, and a Spot or a Fluffy is not for everyone. But if you feel a pet may be a welcome fit in your life, he or she can be a wonderful way to help your brain be its best.

Chapter 8

THE SPIRITUAL BRAIN

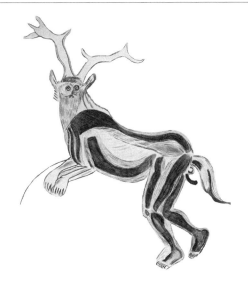

*The Sorcerer, a prehistoric cave painting interpreted to be a
great spirit, master of animals, or deity of good hunting, and believed
to be humans' first-ever depiction of a spiritual essence.*

—CAVE OF THE TROIS-FRÈRES,
ARIÈGE, FRANCE, 13,000 BC
(SKETCH BY HENRI BREUIL)

You are a vibrant, multidimensional being, and in order to live with your
best possible brain, it is important to not only focus on the biological,
psychological, and social but also the spiritual. In this chapter, we address the
human spiritual side with the intent to help you optimize brain health through

this powerful dimension. Engaging in spirituality, attached to religion or not, is fundamental for many people, and most of the data show that doing so can be enormously beneficial for the brain on a number of levels. But first we'll make a distinction between spirituality and religion. In the simplest health-related terms, spirituality is about meaning and purpose. It is about your relationship with yourself and with the outside world. For some, this means observing a religion that provides a foundation, structure, and rituals that facilitate spirituality. For others, it is doing something creative, volunteering in the community, or learning a meditation practice.

The important thing is that you take the time to explore what will make your spiritual brain thrive. Perhaps you enjoyed religious services at one time but then moved to a new town and never took the time to find a new place of worship. Or maybe you had a bad experience with religion and would prefer to find another path for your spiritual brain but haven't made this a priority. We are here to tell you that your brain's health depends on it. Based on our research, we believe that spirituality is as important to health as exercise, and like exercise, most of us do not get enough of it. As a starting point, ask yourself: What's my religious belief system? What are the things that give me a sense of purpose and meaning? Are there things I've wanted to explore like meditation or an art class, but just haven't made the time for? It is important to understand where you are in terms of the religious and the spiritual. Depending on whether you are religious and spiritual, spiritual but not religious, religious but not spiritual, or neither spiritual nor religious, you might seek different approaches to engaging this part of yourself.

You may hold a traditional religious belief system such as Judaism, Catholicism, Buddhism, or Islam. Or you may take a more agnostic approach with some notion of a spiritual perspective but nothing formal. We also emphasize for those who consider themselves to be atheists that there is almost no limit to the ways in which you can connect to your spiritual selves, with humanism being just one of them. With these different perspectives in mind, let's dive into understanding how religiosity and spirituality affect your brain health and how you can find ways to infuse them into your plan for an optimal brain.

THE RELIGIOUS

We'll discuss religion itself as a form of spirituality since there is substantial research. If you have a strong religious belief system, there is great news for you in the research. A growing number of studies have shown that people who are most religious or go to religious services as often as possible tend to derive specific brain health from those activities. For example, one study showed that the people who attended church most often had the lowest rates of anxiety and depression.[1] This appeared to hold true regardless of gender or age.

Some exciting work by Dr. Lisa Miller at Columbia University has focused on adolescents, who are particularly prone to mental health concerns such as anxiety, distress, substance abuse, and suicide. Her research has shown that adolescents who engaged more so than their counterparts in a specific religious tradition were better protected against those kinds of mental health conditions.[2] Adolescents who attended church most often had lower risks and rates for depression, substance abuse, and suicide. Hence, connecting struggling adolescents to religious and spiritual practices might be quite beneficial for them.

Of course, whenever we talk about engaging in religious practices, it almost goes without saying that we always mean engaging in those practices that resonate with you. We would never suggest making yourself go to services that are against your belief system or making anyone else, including adolescents, do so. In fact, the data are clear that forcing beliefs and practices on others not only doesn't help them; often it causes them harm. And we would never tell an atheist that because the research shows going to church is beneficial means that he or she ought to go too. This would be ridiculous advice, and there are of course many other ways atheists can engage in spirituality. If you have always held a strong sense of faith, it might be particularly helpful to stay as actively engaged as possible with your church, synagogue, or mosque. As with everything else we have described in this book, all things must be tailored to what makes sense for you individually.

Work by Dr. Harold Koenig has also shown that adults derive sufficient and substantial benefits from engaging in religious activities.[3] Adults who attend church most often, a reasonable marker for how religious a person is, tend to do better in terms of their overall brain health. They have lower levels of anxiety and depression than those who do not attend church frequently. And since we know that anxiety and depression are particularly bad for the brain, helping to reduce those levels early in life is likely to lead to long-term brain health over the course of a lifetime.

An important question that has been the focus of much of our own research is: What is the main ingredient or ingredients associated with religious activities that confer brain health? What we mean by this is that when you go to church, for example, there are many different elements that can have a beneficial effect on your brain. As we will explore in chapter 12, meditation and prayer tend to have substantial benefits for the brain's functions. If you go to church in order to spend a fair amount of time praying or meditating, that practice in and of itself is likely to provide a benefit for your brain. Engaging in various religious holidays, beliefs, and rituals can be uplifting and give a sense of meaning and purpose in life, as well as be quite beneficial for maintaining good brain health. Research studies have shown that people who are most optimistic also have the overall best levels of health.[4] If a sense of meaning and purpose confers a sense of optimism and good things happening in the future, it is reasonable to expect a similar improvement in overall health, including brain health. In that regard, the positive emotional responses that people derive from religion—joy, happiness, love, compassion—will all result in reduced stress and anxiety and improved functioning of the brain.

Perhaps one of the most important beneficial elements of religious practices is the social engagement. As we have noted, people with the most social support are known to have the highest levels of physical and mental health. The ability to have others support you through various challenges in life clearly confers a great deal of benefit to your brain. And when it comes to coping with various life stressors such as a serious physical illness like cancer or heart disease, a life challenge such as the death of a spouse or child, or a financial stressor such as losing a job, having social support from a community is extremely helpful. A religious community can help you cope and deal with the various problems you are facing as well as help you in solving them.

Perhaps one of the most intriguing possibilities for religion with respect to brain health is that it provides a way of reducing what might be called ontological anxiety.[5] This goes beyond mere meaning and purpose in life to providing an explanation for how the world works and how we are supposed to interact with it. Our brain functions best, and is most comfortable, when we feel that we understand the world around us and have a sense of what we need to do in order to survive and thrive. Religion provides such a perspective. By reducing this fundamental ontological anxiety, the brain can work more optimally. Of course, trying to measure this in any kind of scientific experiment is almost impossible. But in terms of how we understand both religion and the brain, this all makes sense. In fact, an early argument in *Why God Won't Go Away*, one of Andy's previous best-selling books, has to do with the important role the brain has in self-maintenance.[6] Some of the brain's primary jobs are to help us maintain who we are, help us interact with the world, and help us survive. It appears that religion maps well onto these processes by giving us an understanding of ourselves, regulating our body's functions through various practices like meditation and prayer, and providing us with a sense of ontological wisdom.

Another important point about religion and the brain involves the data that validate the conclusion: the more ways we activate our brain, the better our brain works. As we said before, if you like to do crossword puzzles, it is great to do them. But it is also important to do other kinds of puzzles, as well as talk to people, exercise, read, and do many other brain-stimulating activities. In one respect, religion can provide a similar diversity of activities. Study, prayer, meditation, social engagement, and various ritual activities all engage the brain in lots of different ways, and as the brain becomes more stimulated, the better all of its functions work. Yet religion can also sometimes become problematic if a person ends up following a narrow set of beliefs, never questions them, or never engages with others who see things differently, which essentially keeps them isolated and provides limited brain engagement.

This leads us to an important discussion about the potentially negative side of religion. While the overwhelming amount of research is pretty rosy, there are times when religion does not fortify the spiritual brain. In addition to those who end up practicing a limited perspective, religion can also encourage racism, sexism, elitism, and outward aggression and hatred toward others.[7] These intense negative emotional reactions can lead to heightened anxiety and stress in the brain that further limit its functions and increase the risk of poorer brain health. For example, individuals who follow religious cults or radical terrorist groups can engage both inwardly and outwardly in destructive behaviors that are seriously problematic for their own brain health and for the world's health collectively.

While there is not a great deal of neuroscientific data on exactly why some people go down these negative paths of religion, it is an important field of future research with the goal of not only understanding how they got there but also of finding ways of helping to redirect them toward more positive paths that foster openness and compassion toward themselves and others. The research has clearly shown that the more open and compassionate we are, the lower are our levels of stress, anxiety, and depression and the better our overall brain health becomes. When religion fosters love and compassion, brain health goes up dramatically. When it instead fosters anger, hatred, and the desire to dominate others, brain health goes down dramatically.

SPIRITUAL BUT NOT RELIGIOUS

Many people choose to not follow specific religious traditions but nevertheless find alternative routes for engaging the spiritual side of their brain. If you are in this category, you may feel a strong connection to the universe or the rest of humanity and try to foster it through various spiritual pursuits such as volunteering at a food bank or building up global awareness. Other spiritual pursuits can include practicing meditation, engaging in spiritual communities such as yoga groups or retreats, or following other spiritual paths through creativity, music, or nature.

The research generally shows that such spiritual paths, much like more formal religious approaches, can be highly beneficial for your brain. Meditation or yoga are the best studied and have repeatedly been shown to result in a variety of changes in brain function that contribute to enhanced cognitive functioning and improved emotional processing. Similarly, any practice or activity that takes your mind away from stressors, helps you feel more connected and grounded with yourself, and makes you feel more connected to the universe and humanity will typically result in a beneficial effect on your brain.

For all of these reasons, engaging your spiritual side can be beneficial to you in weaving together your best brain possible. Certainly seek out as many of these activities as you feel comfortable with and try to make them a regular part of your life, always remembering that the more different kinds of engagement you practice, the better off you are. Doing something creative, taking hikes in the woods, helping out a charity, or trying to save the environment can all be great spiritually oriented activities that lead to better brain health.

BENEFITS, NOT BELIEFS

If you consider yourself to be neither spiritual nor religious, perhaps you not only disagree with the primary tenets of any given religion, but you also do not perceive something more spiritual or find specific meaning in anything outside of the physical world. Nonetheless, the data show that doing the kinds of activities we are calling "spiritual"—even if you use a different word to describe them, including being in nature or expressing your creative side—can still be beneficial.

Our work with a mindfulness-based art therapy program revealed not only reductions in anxiety and depression but also significant changes in the brain itself.[8] Art and creativity have dramatic effects on the brain's functions. This occurs whether you are actively in the process of creation—painting a picture or writing music—or passively viewing an art piece or listening to a song. The more you go to art exhibits, music presentations, or, better still, use your own creative powers, the more you stimulate different parts of your brain. But if you do go to a concert or art museum, make sure that you are fully engaged there. By this we mean it is important to try to fully appreciate what you are doing and what that creative expression means to you. In a similar manner, if you are religious, it is not just going to church that is important, but rather that you fully engage in being at church. Simply sitting there will not confer much benefit to your brain. Actively engaging in prayer, rituals, and listening and considering in-depth the words of a sermon are all important ways to help enable your brain to function more effectively. Again, the more you can fully engage in creative, life-enhancing activities, the better your brain will function.

This includes engaging in humanistic and compassionate activities such as donating to causes you believe in or helping others in need, which can be highly rewarding to your brain health as well as to society. For example, studies have shown that performing charitable acts can enhance brain function. A study that used functional brain scans showed that when people open-heartedly donated money rather than feeling coerced into giving it, they activated the "feel-good" centers of the brain that are involved with the release of dopamine.[9] Such an effect, if done repeatedly, can create a brain that is filled with positive thoughts and positive emotions—all good things for healthfulness. In fact, when you help others, you help not only your brain but their brains as well. By providing food, comfort, and other necessities, you help them build a foundation that supports their brain and helps it to function as well as possible.

SPIRITUALITY CHANGES THE BRAIN, SOMETIMES MORE THAN DRUGS DO

To fully emphasize the importance of religion and spirituality in the context of creating optimal brain health, we share the fairly extensive amount of research our team has performed over the past twenty years that has included observing the effects directly through brain imaging studies. Our earliest work looked at practices such as meditation and prayer. One of our studies used brain scans to observe Franciscan nuns while they performed a centering prayer[10] a highly meditative technique in which you bring your full attention to a specific prayer or phrase from the Bible. It is not a matter of simply repeating that phrase, but reflecting over and over on its meaning, in general and as it relates to you personally. The ultimate goal of the practice is to experience being more deeply connected to, or even at one with, God.

For this study, nuns came to our laboratory in order to perform the practice while we scanned their brains. We used a specific technique, single photon emission computed tomography (SPECT imaging). This technique required us to inject a small amount of a radioactive tracer into a participant's arm at a particular moment: the peak of their centering prayer practice. We put an intravenous catheter in each nun's arm long before they engaged in the practice so that when we injected the tracer, it would not disturb their concentration at all—they remained in the lab with Bible in hand while doing their practice and we injected them at a specific time. After each completed her centering prayer, we moved her into the scanner to take a picture of her brain. The scan would tell us what her brain was doing during the prayer and at the time of the injection.

The results were quite remarkable, some of which you can see in the brain imaging figures titled Prayer and the Brain in the color photography section. There were two main findings. The first was that their frontal lobes showed increased activity and their parietal lobes decreased activity. This made a great deal of sense based on what the centering prayer was meant to do. The frontal lobe becomes activated when a person focuses attention on anything, and these nuns were intensely focused on a particular prayer or phrase from the Bible, so focusing on a prayer would also cause an increase in their frontal lobe activity. This is precisely what we saw. Perhaps more important, their parietal lobe activity decreased. The parietal lobe typically takes sensory information and helps us create a spatial sense of ourselves and an understanding of how our self relates to the rest of the world. So if increasing activity in the parietal lobe helps you establish your sense of self, when you lose that sense of self and feel instead intimately connected—meaning at one with the world or God—you can expect a decrease of activity in the parietal lobe. Again, this is precisely what we saw. Please see the brain imaging figures titled Sense of Connectedness and the Brain in the color photography section for evidence of this.

This loss of a sense of self is a fascinating and important phenomenon generally associated with spiritual practices and has an interesting effect on brain health. It is common to think that brain health is best preserved by focusing more and more on your self instead of letting it go. After all, if your self goes away, how can you maintain its health? But the data suggest that by losing the sense of self and feeling connected with the rest of the world, we increase our sense of compassion and love, and reduce our overall levels of stress to boot. In this way, the experience of losing oneself can actually be highly advantageous for brain health. The only exceptions to this might be for those with severe disorders such as schizophrenia who already cannot adequately hold on to their sense of self.

In the context of brain health, these developments may be quite important. The ability to increase your frontal lobe activity is essential for helping your attention and concentration. Thus, repeatedly doing a spiritual practice like a centering prayer can be beneficial to helping the brain apply concentration in other areas, such as in solving a conflict at work, taking a final examination, or learning a new trade. In addition, the frontal lobe helps regulate emotional responses. Higher frontal lobe activity helps us reduce our stress and anxiety, and this is exactly what other studies exploring the effects of prayer have found. For example, we did a study of Catholics performing the rosary.[11] Those who performed the rosary regularly were found to have much lower levels of stress and anxiety compared to those who did not. An important caveat, as we mentioned before, is that we would recommend the rosary only to those who believe in it. It would not make sense to recommend doing the rosary to a Muslim simply because we have data that show it can reduce anxiety. However, we can extrapolate from this finding and suggest that Muslims might perform a recited devotional known as the *dhikr* as a way to help reduce their stress and anxiety.

Another fascinating study we performed was with a group of Pentecostal Christians who practiced speaking in tongues (glossolalia).[12] This unique practice that arose from the Pentecostal tradition is one in which believers make vocalizations that sound like language yet are not related to any specific language. For these individuals, this ritual is incredibly powerful and has a great deal of religious and spiritual meaning. Churches that perform it often have interpreters charged with helping people understand the meaning and purpose of what is happening during the speaking in tongues. Watching those in our study perform speaking in tongues was quite remarkable. These completely normal-looking individuals with jobs, families, and otherwise regular lives entered into this ecstatic experience with tears rolling down their faces. They were in a completely different state of consciousness. For the period of time that they were speaking in tongues, it was almost impossible to disturb them because they were so intensely involved in the moment. But five to ten minutes after the practice was over, they were back to their everyday selves. Neurologically, this practice is associated with specific changes in brain function, including activity in their frontal and parietal lobes, which regulate their emotional responses and abilities to think cognitively.

There are also a few anecdotal reports in the medical literature about people undergoing a psychosis-like experience during their intense practices of meditation or prayer. Like everything else in this book, there is no one-size-fits-all practice. However, barring those with significant mental health concerns, spiritual practices appear to be highly advantageous for those who abide by them.

BASELINE   MEDITATION

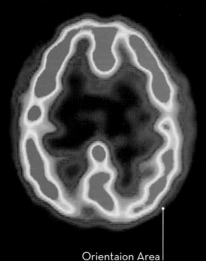 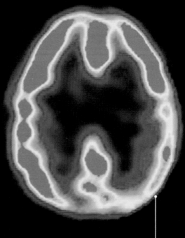

Orientaion Area   Orientaion Area

Meditation and the Brain. SPECT brain scan results of baseline function (left) and
those during Tibetan Buddhist meditation (right) show a decrease in activity in the
parietal lobes. These findings are consistent with a loss of a sense of self that is
normally generated by the parietal lobe and with a feeling of oneness characteristic
of meditation.

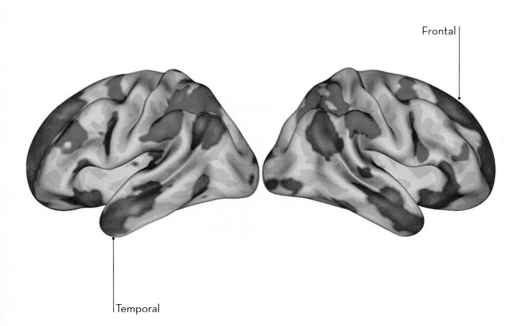

Frontal

Temporal

Vibro-Auditory Therapy for Insomnia. Functional MRI brain scans show significant differences in connectivity between the pre-treatment and post-treatment conditions with vibro-auditory therapy for insomnia. The results indicate increased functional connectivity in the temporal lobes (left) and in the frontal areas (right) consistent with improved sleep, concentration, and memory. Areas of decreased connectivity in some of the central regions are also consistent with better modulation of motor and sensory activity that is a result of improved sleep.

BASELINE

PRAYER

Frontal

Frontal

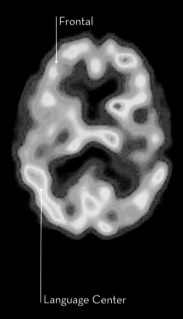

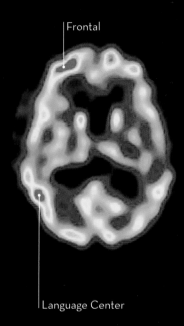

Language Center

Language Center

Prayer and the Brain. SPECT brain scans of a Franciscan nun show her baseline brain function (left) and increased activity (right) during prayer in the frontal lobe and also in the language area near the junction of the temporal and parietal lobes. These findings are consistent with increased mental concentration and use of language during prayer.

BASELINE

CONNECTEDNESS

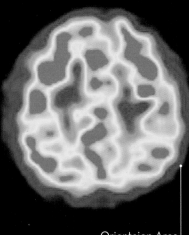

Orientaion Area

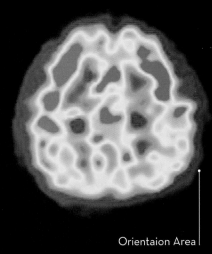

Orientaion Area

Sense of Connectedness and the Brain. SPECT brain scan results of baseline brain function (left) and those during prayer (right) show decreased activity in the parietal lobes. These findings are consistent with a loss of a sense of self that is normally generated by the parietal lobe and with a sense of connectedness with God or other deity during prayer.

TRAUMA
PRE-TREATMENT

TRAUMA
POST-TREATMENT

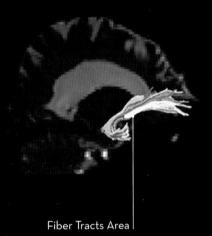

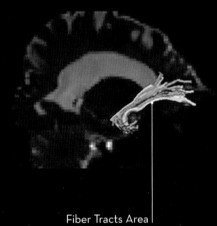

Fiber Tracts Area

Fiber Tracts Area

Trauma Recovery Treatment. Diffusion tensor imaging MRI brain scans of a patient with cancer-related traumatic stress pre-treatment (left) and post-treatment results using the Neuro Emotional Technique (right) show an increase in fiber tract connectivity between the frontal lobes and the amygdala. This increase indicates improved patient control over emotional reactivity.

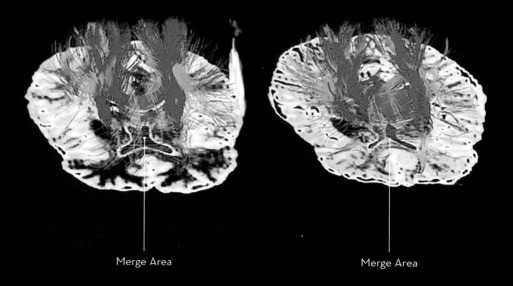

CREATIVE

HIGHLY
CREATIVE

Merge Area

Merge Area

Creativity and the Brain. MRI brain scans of a normally creative person (left) and a highly creative person (right) show a significant difference in fiber tracts of the corpus callosum that merge the left and right hemispheres. Creativity may involve more connectivity between the two hemispheres to allow for a heightened combination of the analytical and artistic sides of the brain.

BASELINE

YOGA

Attention Area

Attention Area

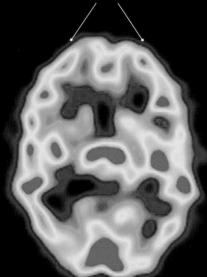

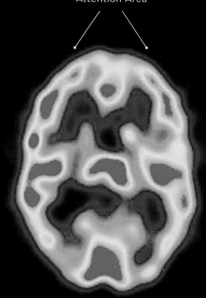

Yoga and the Brain. SPECT brain scan results of baseline brain function (left) and those during yoga (right) show an increase in activity in the frontal lobe. These findings are consistent with increased mental concentration and relaxation during yoga.

BASELINE

SUPPLEMENT

Temporal

Temporal

Natural Supplement for Multiple Sclerosis Treatment. Fluorodeoxyglucose (FDG) PET scan of a patient with multiple sclerosis pre-treatment (left) and post-treatment results (right) after receiving two months of N-acetylcysteine (NAC) show an increase in metabolism in the temporal lobes. These findings are consistent with improvements in cognition and attention.

PART TWO

Healing Systems

Chapter 9

MENTAL FITNESS THROUGH PHYSICAL FITNESS

To keep the body in good health is a duty . . .
otherwise we shall not be able to keep our mind strong and clear.

—Buddha, circa 500 BC

Physical exercise is one of the best kinds of exercise you can do for your brain. Over the past thirty years, a large amount of research has demonstrated the incredible value that physical exercise has for helping the brain stay healthy. Of course, there are many types of physical exercise, and we will explore which options might be best for you. But the bottom line is that the more you move, the better your brain will be.

The positive effect that physical exercise has on your brain comes from various aspects of the exercises you do. Aerobic exercise helps increase blood flow and oxygenation to your body and brain.[1] Thus, the more you can get your heart rate up and your breathing up, the more blood and oxygen you get to your brain; anaerobic or strength training exercises help regulate the cells of your muscles and body, thus enhancing your overall functioning. And as you likely already know, exercise is a wonderful way to relieve stress.

The effects of exercise also extend to many physiological processes, including how genes are expressed, how neurons grow, and how the autonomic nervous systems is balanced. It also decreases inflammation and oxidative stress, which, as we have already discussed, is detrimental to the brain. Exercise affects a number of neurotransmitters and hormones as well. All of these effects result in a body and brain that run more effectively and efficiently. As we will explore in more detail, exercise also has benefits for cognition, anxiety and depression management, sleep, coping skills, and social interactions.

Like with everything we have explored so far, exercise must be considered in the light of moderation and balance. In fact, there is some evidence to suggest that extreme forms of exercise may be detrimental to the brain and body. But more about that later.

EXERCISE PROGRAMS

Aerobic exercises come in many forms. The simplest of all is walking, and it is quite effective. We encourage all of our patients to walk as much as possible. When you are at work, walk to lunch or walk up several flights of stairs to your next meeting. When you are at home, walk to the market if you can or just take a walk . Walking is an excellent aerobic exercise and is low impact so it is easy on your joints. If you can tolerate more intense exercise, do more of the things you enjoy, such as taking dance classes, biking, or swimming, all of which can give an excellent aerobic workout. As we age, activities that have a lot of high impact like running and jumping can be too stressful on the joints of the hip and lower limbs. which can lead to injury or chronic pain such as arthritis and other joint deterioration. Better alternatives include swimming and cross-country skiing, both of which engage your arms and legs at relatively low impact. Biking can also be a wonderful exercise, but care must be taken to ride in a setting that is safe such as on bike paths, and it is important to wear a helmet and make sure you have plenty of drinking fluid with you. Swimming provides a great cardiovascular work out and is sometimes referred to as the perfect exercise because it is low impact yet tones the entire body. The downside is that not everyone has easy access to a pool.

There are also many options for structured training programs such as aerobics classes, cycling and spinning classes, and core workout programs Any one of these can be beneficial. The important thing is to find one that works best for you and ideally is something you look forward to doing. If you love to go bike riding, that can be great exercise for you. But if you don't feel comfortable on a bike, you won't do it consistently since it is not associated with a positive emotion, and you'll likely drop out. Or consider swimming or walking. And if you live in colder climates, cross-country skiing, snowshoeing, and even downhill skiing are excellent forms of exercise.

Not only does aerobic exercise bring more oxygen and blood flow to your brain; it reduces your risk of heart disease, stroke, and, most important, obesity. Any of these medical conditions can lead to significant damage to your brain. Thus, to have an optimal brain, do your best to reduce the risk of these conditions occurring.

Strength training is more anaerobic, though it can still be helpful for overall health. Lifting weights can help increase your muscle tone and be a great stress reliever. If you are trying this type of exercise for the first time, take care to work with someone who can train you appropriately and make sure that you do not injure yourself.

You can also benefit from forms of exercise derived from ancient practices. For example, many people like moving meditations such as yoga and tai chi. These incorporate slow body movements, balance, and stretching postures to enhance the body's function, but more specifically to promote serenity and spiritual experiences. Some excellent research shows that these practices can be beneficial for improving brain function.[2] And because of their often mild nature, they can be helpful for people with a number of psychiatric or neurological conditions, including older individuals. Yoga has been shown to be beneficial for depression and anxiety, as well as to help with balance, mobility, and quality of life for those with neurodegenerative disorders and brain injury.[3]

THE BRAIN BENEFITS OF EXERCISE

Aerobic exercise has also been demonstrated to be a potent inducer of neuroplasticity.[4] In other words, exercise can stimulate the brain to produce more neurons and more neural connections in support of its overall functioning. It is also important to note that exercise-induced neuroplasticity is not restricted to young people. It can be effective into advanced old age.

Studies have shown that regular physical exercise is even associated with larger brains, particularly in areas such as the frontal lobe and hippocampus, which are involved in attention and memory, respectively.[5] Interestingly, the effect of exercise on your brain is not just where the neurons are, the gray matter, but also in the white matter that contains the connecting fibers among neurons. While many forms of exercise can cause neuroplasticity, aerobic exercise appears to be the most effective. Overall, it is beneficial to develop an exercise program that emphasizes aerobic activity while including some resistance, or anaerobic, exercises as well.

Studies have also detailed how this neuroplasticity happens on a physiological level. Exercise results in the release of a family of molecules that are involved in neurogenesis. It seems that the stress of exercise can be a good thing by stimulating the brain to develop. For instance, the brain-derived neurotrophic factor (BDNF) molecule is significantly increased as a result of exercise.[6] In addition, other molecules that stimulate blood vessels to grow and genes to be expressed in an increasing amount are associated with exercise. Even resistance exercise may be involved in releasing similar factors in the brain that help it develop and increase its connections.

Exercise also improves brain function by increasing the amounts of a variety of neurotransmitters. These chemicals, such as serotonin and dopamine, have widespread effects on cognitive and emotional processes. For example, serotonin has been shown to improve mood, memory, sexuality, and attention. A precursor molecule, tryptophan, is an amino acid that becomes increasingly available to the brain during exercise. The implication is that exercise leads to higher amounts of serotonin in the brain. In fact, doing an exercise such as swimming for thirty minutes a day has been shown to increase serotonin in the cerebral cortex and brain stem, increases that can last a week after discontinuing the exercise.[7]

Exercise has also been shown to increase dopamine levels in a variety of brain areas that are involved in your motor, emotional, and cognitive processes. It is likely that part of the way exercise benefits your brain is by boosting dopamine levels so that it works more effectively. And since dopamine is a feel-good molecule, exercise elevates your mood, which also has benefits for your overall brain function. Endorphins are another feel-good molecule released during exercise.

Research to date has pointed to other ways exercise has a measurably positive effect on cognitive processes. Numerous studies have correlated increased levels of aerobic fitness with higher cognitive health as measured by higher IQ scores, better academic achievement, preserved cognitive function with aging, and lower rates of dementia. It seems that exercise is good for your cognitive health no matter how old you are or what your cognitive baseline might be.

Although we explore how exercise has a substantial impact on various brain-based maladies such as anxiety and depression in more detail in upcoming chapters, it is worth mentioning here that a large number of studies have documented how valuable exercise can be for patients with a wide variety of physical and mental conditions. Even people with significant medical problems benefit from exercising, although usually this has been seen with lower-impact exercises such as yoga or walking. So carefully design your exercise program for your unique needs and limitations by starting slowly and working up to a good level of aerobic exercise, usually at least thirty to forty-five minutes a day, five or six days a week. You can work in a similar amount of resistance training to balance with the aerobic training, so maybe do three days of each, alternating days. Check with your doctor to make sure that whatever you choose to pursue is safe based on your health, particularly your heart and lungs. Your brain and body were designed to move and to be agile, both of which are essential for maintaining adequate tone, circulation, and vibrancy.

Chapter 10

THE EFFECTS OF STRESS AND STRESS REDUCTION ON BRAINPOWER

The trouble with the rat race is that even if you win, you're still a rat.

—LILY TOMLIN, 1977

Effective navigation of stress is a critical component of weaving the fabric for your best brain. Of course, all stress isn't bad, and your brain, as well as every other organ in your body, requires some level of stress for proper development. Only by using and even pushing yourself to solve problems, explore the world, and interact with others can the neural connections that support these functions form and strengthen. However, too much stress on any organ, including the brain, can be detrimental. Just like weaving a tapestry, if you pull the threads too tight, they will break, and if they are too loose, the whole tapestry will fall apart. This means that you have to apply just the right amount of tension throughout the entire process. The brain is exactly the same. In society today, there is excessive toxic stress that is unhealthy and even damaging to the brain. The good news is that there are highly effective ways, supported by science, to deal with that stress that are easy to implement in your daily life. Our goal is to help you recognize how the negative stressors in your life are weighing you down and empower you with a set of tools that will help you achieve optimal brain function.

STRESS THAT IS GOOD FOR THE BRAIN

To delve into this question a bit more deeply, it is helpful to first recognize that neurons work by connecting with other neurons in the brain. These connections occur between the axon, the part of the nerve cell that extends toward the next neuron in the system, and the dendrites on the next neuron that receives the signal. Thus, two neurons interact because the axon from one neuron touches one or more subsequent neurons and then releases a signal, usually in the form of a molecule such as dopamine or serotonin.

Children have an overabundance of connections between different nerve cells, and for this reason, they have overactive imaginations. Sometimes there are neural connections that are not useful. For example, it is important to have the neural connection that corresponds to 1 + 2 = 3. But if a neural connection says 1 + 2 = 4, that is obviously a connection you don't need. As you grow and develop, especially through stress (perhaps when you were young, your classmates laughed at you because you got the 1 + 2 math problem wrong), you will cut back on connections you don't need. Various neurons and interneurons help this process occur.

The best way to think about the process of forming connections and losing connections is through two common phrases. The first phrase is, "Neurons that fire together, wire together," which means that the more you use a specific neural connection, the stronger it becomes. So if you keep using the neural connection that supports 1 + 2 = 3, that will be the information you remember. The second phrase is, "Use it or lose it." Neural connections you don't need become weaker and eventually fade away if you no longer use them. This overall process enables you to interweave connections in your brain as effectively as possible. It helps you learn new information and adapt to new environments, and it also helps you create a specific set of ideas and beliefs that you use to navigate through the world. Hence, good stress for the brain is the kind that you control and implement to increase learning and reinforce brain pathways for specific skills that help you live a better life.

STRESS THAT IS BAD FOR THE BRAIN

If your system is overloaded, your brain will begin to struggle greatly. The defining of this stress as good or bad has to do with the types of stressors you are under. The things that register in your brain as a threat to your survival and well-being and that are not in your immediate control, such as a job that feels tenuous (the threat of losing your income), a pandemic (the threat of losing people you care about or the threat to your own passing), or political battles (the threat that you won't be fairly represented by elected officials), threaten your safety in some way, and that experience links to how well you manage to survive. The problem is that too many of us juggle a myriad of these types of stressors and the thing that puts us over the top is the sense that we have no control over it all. So when the stress response occurs, several important things happen. For one, a part of your brain, the amygdala, typically becomes more active in pointing out to you that there is something wrong that you need to pay attention to. Interestingly, the amygdala can become active for both good or bad things. But it is most notoriously known as the center for anxiety and stress because it becomes particularly active when confronted with such feelings.

When the amygdala becomes active, it interacts with another structure, the hypothalamus, which regulates your autonomic nervous system. In the face of stress, it elicits the famed fight-or-flight response. This response increases your heart rate and blood pressure and readies your body for action against the stress.

Ultimately you have an adaptive function that is highly useful for keeping you alive in a world with a great many dangers. It is also important to note that the amygdala, in conjunction with the hippocampus, writes information into your memory. Specifically, events that trigger your stressful response elicit a strong memory so that you can be better prepared to avoid whatever that danger is in the future.

In addition to activating the arousal part of your autonomic nervous system, your brain also tells your adrenal glands to release cortisol and adrenaline. These hormones, which help to activate other areas of your body and brain, also can have a negative impact if the brain is exposed to them over a prolonged period of time. This has been observed in animals raised in stressful environments: they are found to have far fewer neural connections than animals raised in enriching environments.[1] Similarly, people who have post-traumatic stress disorder have been found to have atrophy (or shrinkage), particularly in the amygdala and hippocampus, compared to those with normal levels of stress in their lives.[2]

Stress and its associated emotions of anxiety, anger, and depression all lead to a similar path of increased stress hormones and an increased response from the autonomic nervous system that over time can be quite detrimental to the brain. Neurons that fire together wire together, making the stress response more automatic. This connection can set up a vicious cycle, where a heightened state makes the brain more vulnerable to a stress response whenever other pressures come along. This can also lead people to engage in behaviors that bring on even more stress and thus make their brain less resilient to stress overall. Behaviors such as overeating, drinking too much alcohol, smoking, or using drugs (both prescription and recreational) can all lead to more stress. We next discuss proven ways of breaking out of this cycle and modifying your reaction to specific stressors so that the stress response is no longer in overdrive and allowing your brain to restore itself and achieve more optimal levels of functioning.

WEAVING A DE-STRESSED BRAIN

You can reduce the amount of stress your brain feels in a number of ways. The most obvious one is to try to eliminate some of the more severe external stressors from your life. Sometimes this is possible. For example, if you are in a stressful job and can find an alternative, that might be the best way to reduce this type of stress. Similarly, if you are in a bad relationship and feel that you can leave, sometimes that can be the most effective way to resolve high stress levels. Of course, those options are not always available. But it is important to take stock of all the ways in which your brain and body perceive stress, identify the ones that are possible to change, and see if implementing those changes helps to reduce your stress to a tolerable level. The goal is to manage all your various levels and causes of stress so they do not interfere with your overall well-being and brain function.

For the external stressors you cannot change, and all of us have some, there are a number of effective ways to adapt your responses to them. As the late, great Lena Horne said, "It's not the load that breaks you down, but the way you carry it." Some of the most powerful approaches are simple to do.

The first is to breathe. You might be saying to yourself, *That's ridiculous. Of course I breathe!* But when you examine how you breathe, you might find that you take short, halting breaths, often holding them in for seconds at a time, and even laboring at it. This is the breathing pattern of someone in a fight-or-flight mode. By taking a couple of moments a day and thinking about how you are breathing, you will notice that simply thinking about it changes it. You probably will then take deeper, more rhythmic breaths as you focus. Next, we suggest you take several deep breaths slowly in and out for sixty seconds; some people like to count up to five during each inhalation and exhalation. You can do this at home, at your desk, in your car, or anywhere else, and it can almost immediately reset your nervous system and help to defuse your stress. You can even try this right before engaging in a stressful activity or event, like giving a presentation or having a difficult conversation with your boss or loved one. This simple breath work will help you relax and enable you to focus more effectively during those encounters. It may even make you function better, so that the potentially stressful situation ends up being a lot easier than you though it would be.

One of the most famous stress reduction techniques is progressive muscle relaxation, and it can be a fun exercise. Do your breath work for about a minute; then go through each muscle group in your body, tense it for a count of five seconds, and relax it while focusing on feeling the stress releasing from those muscles. Starting from the top, tense your facial muscles, then your neck, your shoulders, upper arms, lower arms, fists, chest, abdomen, rear end, thighs, calves, feet, and finally toes. Hold each for five seconds as tightly as you can without it being overly uncomfortable, and then release. After doing this exercise for about three to five minutes, you will notice an intense feeling of relaxation in your body.

More complex approaches typically involve developing strategies for stress reduction. Some include more formal types of psychotherapy. Being able to talk to a counselor or psychiatrist can be helpful at working through stressors in your life, finding solutions, and resolving those situations. For example, cognitive behavioral therapy (CBT) helps modify thoughts and behaviors in ways that systematically reduce anxiety and depression. An important point about CBT is that it helps address specific types of stressors and processes through them. For instance, it can be life changing to recontextualize a specific difficult event and learn a reaction that is similar to a positive reaction you have had to other rewarding events you have encountered before. While progressive muscle relaxation or breathing exercises can reduce your stress level immediately, having different ways of responding to stressors at the onset is invaluable.

A popular technique, made famous by Jon Kabat-Zinn, is the Mindfulness-Based Stress Reduction program (MBSR),[3] which has been shown to be highly successful at reducing stress and anxiety. This meditation-based program runs over eight weeks, meeting once a week in small groups. A primary focus of it is learning to be present in the moment, nonjudgmentally, which allows for the mental space to appraise stressors more objectively. The MBSR program has been widely tested across populations with illness and those with wellness. Whether coping with a disease or a dysfunctional relationship, mindfulness can be highly empowering and effective. We recently saw a cancer survivor in our clinic who was distressed about some musculoskeletal pains she was having. Although she was assured they were benign, and this logically made sense to her, every time she experienced them, her brain went to a place where she imagined they were instead bone metastases and then she would have a severe stress reaction. The MBSR program helped her to not immediately judge the sensations in her body, allowing her to have a response that was more consistent with the reality of the situation. The effect this has had on her quality of life is incredible.

We have found that the MBSR program works exceptionally well for many of our patients across the board. The published research we have done shows that mindfulness helps rewire the brain, particularly the amygdala, so that it is no longer hyperreactive to stressors.[4] And our most recent research showed that this program helps whether you are young or old.[5] That's because the brain has adaptive mechanisms we are only beginning to understand. Our research showed that the brains of elderly individuals responded well to the MBSR program and in fact changed their brains to be more similar to the brains of younger populations. Contrary to the popular saying, it is never too late to teach an old dog new tricks.

Kirtan Kriya is another meditation practice we described on pages 65–66. It is a basic meditation using repetitive sound. Our study of older individuals practicing this technique showed that they had significant reductions in stress, anxiety, and depression.[6] These were associated with changes in their brain, particularly in the frontal lobes and limbic system, which modulate emotional reactions.

As far as other practices go, each has its own potential benefits and pitfalls. It is important for you to explore many of them, to see which are consistent with your own beliefs and goals. Once you decide which appeal to you, t try them out for a period of time to see if you feel your stress levels have improved. You can then use the one or two that work best for you. Many other meditation techniques also help reduce stress and anxiety and generally help with coping better. Interestingly, most studies of practices such as tai chi, yoga, mindfulness, transcendental meditation, and Kirtan Kriya to name a few, reveal that all of them can work. It is just a matter of finding which one works best for you.

An exciting new intervention is the Neuro Emotional Technique (NET), which combines cognitive restructuring, acupressure and a form of exposure therapy to change the way people respond to significant stressors in their life. In the study we performed with cancer patients, we found they went from stress levels of an 8 or 9 out of 10 to a 1 or 2 after just five sessions. The brain imaging figures titled Trauma Recovery Treatment in the color photography section offer evidence of the benefits that NET can offer. Importantly, the advanced brain scans performed before and after NET showed that the participants had changed the way their brains functioned. For example, the amygdala no longer reacted in the same way to stressful situations. We also looked at the communication pathways of their brains, which is essentially how the brain talks to itself, and found significant differences after going through NET, none of which were observed in the control group. We discovered in this study that the brain's cerebellum is important in traumatic memories and that the connections between the cerebellum and the amygdala changed dramatically after the NET program. This had never been observed before according to scientific literature. We found that these changes were associated with the decrease in their stress and anxiety levels.

DIET, NUTRITION, AND SUPPLEMENTS

While most people consider stress management to be based on various related cognitive, behavioral, and emotional programs, in integrative medicine we also recognize the profound importance of diet and nutrition. If you do not eat a healthy diet, you are more likely to experience stronger stress. The reason for this is multifaceted. First, your brain needs essential vitamins and nutrients to function as optimally as possible. If your brain is deficient in any of these, its processes will be suboptimal and its resilience to stress will be diminished, so your brain will be more easily overwhelmed by external stressors. This is why making sure you have a healthful diet that provides the required nutrients is essential. If eating a diverse, plant-based diet is a challenge for you, consider taking a multivitamin. But even with that, the foundation of your nutrition must come from food, and this must remain your focus. We recommend the diet in *Tapestry of Health* (one of Dan and Dr. Anthony Bazzan's previous books).

Regarding supplemental vitamins relevant to stress, some people prefer to take them individually versus as a multivitamin. A number of B vitamins, for example, are important for many different cellular processes in the brain and body. And although taking high doses of B vitamins is not a treatment for stress and anxiety, making sure that you have the recommended amounts every day does help your brain function optimally. It is ideal to find a B-complex supplement that contains a variety of the B vitamins, including thiamin (B_1), riboflavin (B_2), niacin (B_3), pantothenic acid (B_5), pyridoxine (B_6), biotin (B_7), folate (B_9), and cobalamin (B_{12}). On average, dosages range from 300 milligrams to about 500 milligrams total, taken once per day. Bottle labels will tell you how much there is of each vitamin relative to the recommended daily allowance by the US Recommended Daily Allowance (USRDA). You probably don't need something more than five times the USRDA, and the closer to the daily amount that is recommended, the better.

Vitamin C helps prevent oxidative damage in your nervous system (oxidative damage can result from a number of toxic, infectious or inflammatory processes that release too much oxygen in and around your cells, ultimately causing injury which in turn can increase stress and anxiety). The average supplement dose ranges from 500 to a 1000 milligrams per day. Vitamin D is an important nutrient that helps the body absorb other vitamins and plays a role in many vital cellular processes. Because sunshine offers the main process through which our body makes vitamin D, most of us in the United States have low vitamin D levels. Taking an oral supplement in the range of 1000 to 3000 international units (IUs) per day is typically recommended. Magnesium is necessary for the absorption and metabolism of vitamin D and is also important for a variety of body functions, including possibly bringing on a calming effect. It might also be helpful for those who have stress-associated headaches. Usually it is taken in doses of 100 to 500 milligrams, but sometimes it can cause loose stools or diarrhea so it is important to start at a low dose and increase as tolerated.

Beyond required micronutrients, there is an important mechanism at play between overall nutrition and stress. Many foods are pro-inflammatory, which means that when you eat them, they increase your body's inflammatory reactions. And since stress also causes inflammation, if you eat high-inflammatory foods, you significantly increase your body's inflammatory load, thus making it less resilient to cope with other stressors. Inflammation also fuels negative mood states like depression and anxiety.

A related study of eleven hundred older people in Greece showed that diets high in sugars and saturated fats, two inflammatory foods, were associated with increased anxiety.[7] A similar study from the Netherlands confirmed that poorer diets were associated with more anxiety, likely because of the increased inflammation.[8] Even worse, this is a setup for another vicious cycle: people who are stressed and anxious frequently eat poorly. They crave-high energy, high-sugar foods, which leads them to a more inflamed, less happy life.

It can be difficult to break these cycles, but in our clinic, we use all of the tools we've discussed to help our patients move past these deleterious situations. A key tool is to help them learn about eating the type of integrative diet we prescribe: one that is plant based, with high amounts of protein and plenty of good fats—omega-3 and -9 fats, which are anti-inflammatory—and low in bad fats—saturated fats in dairy and meat, which are pro-inflammatory. A diet high in anti-inflammatory fiber and low in pro-inflammatory processed foods also helps build more resilience to stress.

NATURAL PRODUCTS AND STRESS

Some natural supplements can also reduce stress. We provide some supportive research based on human studies, but it is still best to always consult with your doctor first to determine if any of these are appropriate and safe for you to use. For example, chamomile, lavender, rhodiola, and gamma-aminobutyric acid (GABA) analogues have all been shown to reduce anxiety and stress. Although these compounds do not necessarily enable you to handle specific stressors more effectively, they can create a calming effect that reduces your body's overall stress reactivity. In conjunction with other mind-body approaches, these natural supplements can be beneficial in an overall stress management program.

GABA is an amino acid and neurotransmitter that helps suppress the brain's reactivity. In fact, it is one of the main inhibitory neurotransmitters in the brain, which means it quiets other neurons. The GABA receptors are also the target of well-known medications such as Valium and Xanax, two common benzodiazepines. Taking a small amount of a GABA supplement—200 to 750 milligrams per day—can help reduce stress levels naturally.[9]

L-theanine is an amino acid found in green tea and other sources. Both animal and human studies have demonstrated its calming effects. The average supplement dose is around a 200 milligram tablet once a day.[10]

As previously noted, omega-3 fish oils are important anti-inflammatories and antioxidants. Their fatty acids also are part of what makes up cell membranes, so these oils are helpful for reducing stress and anxiety. The average supplement dose may contain up to 3000 milligrams per day of combined eicosapentaenoic acid (EPA), alpha-linolenic acid (ALA), and docosahexaenoic acid (DHA).

Many herbal remedies have been used to relieve stress and anxiety. A number of these are referred to as *adaptogens* since they enable the brain to adapt better to the environment and stressors. Mostly they work by affecting specific neurotransmitter systems involved in the stress response or by helping reduce inflammation in the body. The clinical data on these are limited, and most of what we know is from nonhuman lab studies that tell us a bit about their mechanism of action.

Ashwagandha (*Withania somnifera*) is an adaptogen that appears to work by reducing the release of cortisol, the main stress hormone in the body. A study of sixty stressed adults found significant reductions in anxiety with a dose of 240 milligrams per day.[11] Bacopa (*Bacopa monnieri*) also reduces cortisol levels, and it may have a neuroprotective effect while reducing anxiety.[12] The average supplement dose is around 300 to 500 milligrams per day as either a single dose or split into two doses.

Chamomile comes from the *Matricaria chamomilla* or *Chamaemelum nobile* species and appears to work on the GABA receptors as well as work as an anti-inflammatory. The average supplement dose ranges from 250 to 500 milligrams per day as a single dose or split into two doses. Of course, many people prefer to drink chamomile tea, which makes for a nice way to benefit from this compound.

Kava kava (*Piper methysticum*) is a plant from the Pacific Islands, where it is used as a traditional calming tonic. As with a number of the compounds we have identified here, it appears to target the GABA receptors to reduce stress and anxiety. The average supplement dose is around 250 milligrams per day as a single dose or split into two doses. However, because there has been some evidence that kava kava may cause liver damage, it is not widely recommended and is best to not use for more than a few weeks at a time.

Lavender (*Lavandula officinalis*) has long been a soothing stress remedy that appears to work by directly reducing neuronal activity or by affecting the serotonin system. Lavender supplements are available as capsules or as an oil, typically with doses of around 400 milligrams per day as a single dose or split into two doses.[13] It is also used in aromatherapy to help reduce anxiety.[14]

Passionflower (*Passiflora incarnata*) is a folk remedy for anxiety that appears to work by affecting the GABA receptors and comes as a supplement or tincture.[15]

The average supplement dose is around 500 milligrams per day as a single dose or split into two doses.

Rhodiola (*Rhodiola rosea*), a plant native to alpine regions, has been used as an adaptogen and calming agent for hundreds of years. It appears to have a unique mechanism that involves activating a number of genes involved in neuronal function and communication. In a trial of eighty mildly anxious patients, it was shown to be effective at reducing anxiety.[16] The average supplement dose per day is around 50 milligrams as a single dose or split into two doses.

A number of formulations are also available that combine these compounds. This is particularly true in Ayurvedic preparations. While these mixtures can be effective, one of the main downsides is that if it works, you don't know if it is one, two, or all of the compounds together that are right for you, so it might be best to work with them one at a time. The other concern with mixtures is that if you develop any side effects or drug interactions, you won't know what is causing them. So when we do consider supplements to help with anxiety or stress, we typically recommend working with them one at a time. Once you find a couple that you like, you might, after a long enough period using them individually to know they all work for you, look for a mixture of those specific compounds.

In the end, some stress is good and necessary for your growth and development. So continually push your nervous systems a bit to learn new things and refine skills that are important to you. However, for many, there is an excess of toxic stress that keeps them in fight-or-flight mode too much of the time, wearing down their brain and lowering their resilience. Hence, incorporating the right tools to combat excess stress is imperative to weaving together your best brain. Mind-body techniques such as mindfulness, breathing exercises, and other therapies can help you keep stress in check. Proper nutrition also is key, which includes getting enough of the right nutrients for optimal brain function and avoiding the ones that increase inflammation and lower resilience.

Chapter 11

ART, MUSIC, AND
THE HEALTHY BRAIN

Creativity takes courage.

—Henri Matisse, circa 1930

Art, music, and creativity are among the most amazing gifts to come from the functions of the human brain; they are also sources for keeping our brain happy and healthy. Virtually everyone loves some type of music or art, and everyone has some creative abilities. Engaging in these gifts is essential for good brain function. And the more you engage your creative and artistic side, the more you strengthen many types of other neural connections that help you in every aspect of your life.

Most research studies exploring the impact of art, music, and creativity on the brain reveal a complex network of structures involved in these activities, which use so many different parts of the brain that they serve as excellent optimizers of the brain's functions. As we have said, the brain has lots of different functions and abilities, and the more you use all of them, the better off you are. Of course, some people tend to focus on one particular creative avenue and may become a concert pianist, a great painter, or a mathematical genius. The more someone focuses on one specific pathway, the stronger and better that particular pathway becomes for them. Yet even people with a singular focus in a seemingly unrelated field can find value in exploring new domains of creativity. For example, Albert Einstein was well known for his love of music. He viewed it to be highly mathematical, and it inspired him to continue exploring his own mathematical abilities. So sometimes turning to domains of creativity can even help you find answers in other areas that you usually focus on.

WEAVING TOGETHER A BETTER BRAIN THROUGH ART

For the purposes of this chapter, when we talk about art, we are referring more often to the visual arts—paintings, sculptures, ceramics, and others that produce something to be looked at. For many people highly engaged in art, their craft is an expression of their spirituality. Creating a work of art or even just looking at art takes them to another level where they feel deeply connected to the world or to God. They may even lose themselves in the experience, much like the spiritual experiences that people who practice religious traditions report.

When it comes to your own appreciation of art, your brain has a tendency to enjoy a sense of wholeness from the experience. The entire composition is something that your brain absorbs, which then evokes an emotional and cognitive response, even if unconsciously, that can affect the way you live in the world. Your brain develops a kind of relationship with the art, and it is that sense of connectedness and oneness that is described as the spiritual component of appreciating art. And while some art, particularly modern art, can have a more fragmented perspective, the fragments still comprise a whole. Intense, peculiar images such as those by Pablo Picasso can evoke a variety of emotions. For example, his painting *Guernica* is known for its elicitation of feelings of horror associated with war.

From a brain health perspective, creating your own art is a fabulous way to express your inner thoughts, experiences, and emotions, even if your skills lag behind Picasso's. A great artist is able to elicit an intended response in others, but for you and the rest of us, there is still a brain-healing quality from doing art just for yourself to express your inner you, regardless of whether anyone else ever sees it. For this reason, art therapy has become a powerful tool in the armamentarium against a wide variety of psychological challenges, including depression, anxiety, and even more severe diseases such as schizophrenia. Empowering others to express their thoughts and feelings through pictures that they cannot express through words is useful not only for them as the creator of art but also for the therapist trying to understand and help them.

Dan has the distinction of performing the first large-scale study of mindfulness-based art therapy that combines a mindfulness-based stress reduction program with a version of art therapy. By creating art mindfully, participants were able to get at their thoughts and feelings in the moment and then reflect on those thoughts and feelings by observing what they had created visually. And by engaging in this process in a nonjudgmental way, we found that it helped them significantly reduce their anxiety and depressive symptoms. It was this study that brought the two of us together because of our mutual interest in seeing the effects of this program not only clinically but neurophysiologically as well.

Using functional MRI, we also studied a subset of patients who underwent the mindfulness-based art therapy program and found significant changes in brain activity, particularly in the amygdala, hippocampus, insula, and caudate nuclei.[1] These are all part of the emotional centers of the brain that help us feel our emotions and respond to them. These brain changes were also correlated with improvements in their anxiety and depression symptoms. The results of the study, shown in the brain imaging figures titled Creativity and the Brain in the color photography section, revealed that art expression, especially combined with mindfulness, is a highly useful way for improving brain health.

Other studies have looked at the impact of art therapy on a variety of conditions. In general, these studies support our own findings that being creative, making and observing art, and participating in art therapy all affect the brain in powerful ways that reduce stress and improve function.

One of the values of art is that it engages the creative parts of the brain, including the parietal and temporal lobes on both the right and left sides. This is important since the left side tends to be more language based, while the right side is more artistic and visual based. Importantly, the data reveal that creating art helps to engage both sides of the brain, and this is perhaps why it is so effective at helping the brain function better.[2] And since most creative processes involve the body and hands, the motor areas of the brain and associated muscles of the body also benefit.

The findings from our own study were even more dramatic than we had expected, which is why we encourage you to find ways of tapping into your artistic side in order to have an optimal brain. There are many different forms of art, so you can almost certainly find one that resonates with you and is enjoyable. Consider drawing, coloring, painting, sculpture, photography, needlepoint, knitting, crocheting, mixed media, or anything else you might like. Importantly, there are also cognitive benefits from this because you typically have to concentrate a fair amount on the artwork at hand, which helps you focus on the moment. In addition, the important hand-eye coordination you develop can be applied to other aspects of your life, including sports, driving, and work-related activities.

This brings us to another interesting point: the paint colors on walls and artwork that adorns them in our workplaces and in our homes can be helpful for maintaining a healthy brain. Research has shown that specific colors such as blues and yellows help people feel calmer and more uplifted.[3] Thus, if you want to surround yourself with an environment that helps you remain calm, you might turn to these colors. If you'd like to be woken up, bright colors such as oranges and reds might be what you are looking for. As with everything else regarding the brain, having an appropriate balance is the best approach, even when it comes to using color in your life. In architecture this can be called *feng shui*, a traditional practice originating in ancient China that claims to use the energy from how a space is arranged to harmonize individuals with that environment through the choice of certain colors, along with shapes, textures, and other elements of art and design.

WEAVING TOGETHER A BETTER BRAIN THROUGH MUSIC

Just like visual art, auditory art—music—is a natural complement to the way your brain works. Research studies looking at neurological electrical activity have revealed that the brain basically works through rhythms. Rhythmic electrical activity is part of how the brain thinks, feels, sleeps, and wakes. Since the brain is awash in rhythms, it appears that the rhythm of sounds taps into its fundamental functions. For example, there are sounds all around us that are essential for us to understand and identify, such as an ambulance siren or a child's laughter. And the brain is particularly adept at being able to distinguish the differences between them, as in the case of a human voice and the differences between calming language and excited language. We hear the distinctions in a tone of voice that have to do with the intensity and the repeatability of the rhythm that the voice and language make.

Your brain has a number of areas involved in processing sounds—in particular, the thalamus, temporal lobe, and auditory cortex. Functional magnetic resonance imaging studies have also documented the pathways involved in our sense of hearing and the impact that different sounds have on brain functions. Slow, rhythmic sounds such as chanting and the sound of the ocean can be relaxing, help your brain achieve a calm state, and even reduce anxiety and stress. But if you're getting ready to do something active like play football, rapid rhythmic sounds such as rock music and rapid drumming can activate your brain.

All kinds of research have observed the effects of music on the brain. For instance, in a hospital operating room, music can help put not only the patient in a calmer state but the surgical team as well.[4] In fact, calm music has been shown to improve surgical outcomes because of the beneficial effect on the brains of both patients and surgeons.

In order to create your own optimal brain program, it is important to recognize what types of music and auditory rhythms you personally enjoy. This is helpful to know especially when it is time to relax (e.g., before going to bed) and when it is good to be aroused (e.g., when you're driving). Different music throughout your day, and even throughout your life, can be essential for guiding your brain through its everyday functions.

While music certainly can help alter your emotional state, it is less clear how much listening to music can improve cognition. A number of years ago, several investigators explored the Mozart effect, particularly in children. In the end, it does not appear that listening to Mozart by itself necessarily makes you smarter, but it probably does make you more relaxed. We have mentioned our earlier study of the Kirtan Kriya meditation practice (please see pages 65–66). Interestingly, the specific one we worked with is a singing meditation, so when we did our study, we compared the meditators to a group of people listening to Mozart concertos.[5] Both groups had improvements in their overall stress and anxiety levels, but the brain areas affected were markedly different. The meditation practice affected some of the higher areas of the brain in the cortex, including the frontal and temporal lobes, while those listening to Mozart tended to activate the auditory cortex and some of the more central, emotional structures of the brain. In some sense, this seems to distinguish between a top-down process in which a person creates the musical rhythms compared to a bottom-up process in which they merely listen to the music.

Actively creating music versus passively listening to it also has some other special effects on the brain. The complex interaction of the hands, sounds, and brain when playing a musical instrument requires a lot of different coordinated processes, because translating musical notes into playing them on an instrument is no easy task. But through practice, you become more skilled and more appreciative of the music you create. You might even take a stab at writing your own music. Engaging in that level of creativity is a great way to exercise your brain.

CREATIVITY AND THE BRAIN

Creative expression, one of the most important qualities that differentiates us from all other animals, can have powerful effects on the brain and even contribute significantly to society. We can create art and music, and science and philosophy, and bridges and skyscrapers. Everything that humanity has done to this point has been through a creative process, and when we look around, we can see how remarkable this aspect of brain function is. All of our technology and science derives from this creativity. All great music and literature similarly comes from it. And even our political and moral systems that guide our everyday lives arise from it. Creativity is fundamental to what it means to be human. And trying to live with an optimal brain means being as creative as possible, thereby using multiple levels of brain functioning at the same time.

All of this adds up to understanding that creative expression is a natural process that we all have to some degree. And while we may not all be da Vincis, Mozarts, or Einsteins, we each have the ability to create for our own lives and for the world we live in that which is meaningful to us. By expressing our innermost thoughts and feelings through creative works, we can get in touch with ourselves and connect more authentically with other people. Doing so taps into the concept of spirituality and offers one of the most brain-healthy things we can do.

Interestingly, it is not yet fully understood how the brain becomes creative. In one way, it is a purposeful process. You can sit down at a piano and compose a piece of music. You can start with a blank canvas and paint a picture. But how exactly does all this happen inside your head? We have performed some of the first imaging research involved in exploring how the brain is creative.[6] In particular, we have looked at highly creative individuals and compared them to normally creative individuals. What we discovered were a number of impressive findings. It seems there are certain areas of the brain that can stimulate creativity, and individuals with larger or more functional areas can have heightened artistic levels. This might help us understand the distinction between the Mozarts of the world and the rest of us. But clearly there is also a continuum of creativity. Yes, we can all create, but some of us are just a little bit creative and others are vastly creative: some of us draw stick figures and some sculpt enduring works like Michelangelo's *David*. Yet from your own brain's perspective, it doesn't really matter how great your creative abilities are. What matters is just fostering your creativity.

One of the things that we noticed in our study of highly creative people was how the two hemispheres in the brain work together when the person is being creative. It makes sense in general that we need both hemispheres since the left one tends to be more analytical and logical, while the right one tends to be more expressive and creative. But when we really need both sides is in creating a particular work of art or piece of music. The reason is that we need the left side to help us establish what concept or pattern we want to develop, while the right side helps us figure out the most interesting way to express it. So when we looked more closely at those people who were the most creative, we found that they had much greater connectivity between their left and right hemispheres, supporting the notion of needing both sides of the brain to be creative.

We also know that the brain has neuroplasticity and can change and develop more over time, which means you can improve your creativity by simply being creative, because this strengthens the pathways between the two sides of your brain. We believe this will help you make your healthiest and most functional brain and that you will enjoy those positive effects with a new ability to navigate through the world. Try taking an art class, learning a musical instrument, or going to an art show or concert. Over time you will see how powerful art, music, and creativity are for your brain and your life.

Chapter 12

THE MEDITATIVE BRAIN

Praying is talking to the Universe. Meditation is listening to it.
—Paulo Coelho, 2017

One of the most important ways to have a highly functioning brain is to exercise it, and one of the best ways to do that appears to be performing one or more meditation-based practices. *Meditation* is a general term that applies to a wide variety of approaches. It can also sometimes have a mixed connotation when people think about meditation in a specifically religious context. However, many meditation practices are agnostic, and there are hundreds of new studies that have looked at all different kinds and have shown their beneficial effects on the brain. Although we have described some of them already, meditation is such a powerful technique that we believe it is important to explore more deeply some of the more commonly used approaches, give you a few specific examples, and help you find a way to create a meditation-based program that works best for you.

WHAT IS MEDITATION?

The basic question about what meditation is doesn't have a simple answer. Many different practices are considered to be meditation even though they might be vastly different from one another. In terms of overall categories, *concentration* or *attention focused* are one of the most common. The general idea is to focus your attention on a particular object, which can be a word, phrase, image, or even a bodily function like your breath. By simply focusing attention on this object, you can start to notice a variety of changes occurring in your brain and even in your body.

A second type of meditation practice refers to the opposite approach: focusing your attention on nothing in particular. These are sometimes referred to as *open monitoring*, or practices in which you attempt to remove all thoughts from your brain and just pay attention to whatever comes into your mind. In general, you do not think about anything in particular but allow your mind to go where it goes and to be aware of that process. However, some of this type of practice also has elements of concentrative practices as well.

A third approach is *moving meditation* such as yoga or tai chi in which a major part of the practice is moving your body while you let your mind observe what you are feeling. Even walking in nature and paying attention to the natural world around you as you move through it can be a kind of moving meditation.

A fourth type of practice might fall into the description of religious practices such as prayer or various rituals associated with specific religious traditions. We discussed these in chapter 8, but it is important to understand that they can also sometimes fit within the realm of meditation.

There are other ways to categorize meditation practices. One expanded approach we developed at the Marcus Institute of Integrative Health focuses not on what you do during the practice but rather on your goal for the practice.[1] Specifically, you might strive for an enhanced emotional state, an enhanced cognitive state, or a null state in which you have emptied your mind. Within these categories are subcategories based on specific traditions and also a set of taxonomic keys, including variables such as whether your eyes are open or closed, you are silent or speaking out loud, sitting or lying down or in other postures; whether there are breath work differences; or even if your goal is to arrive at some metaphysical knowledge. If you are interested in pursuing meditation to high levels, these additional descriptors might become important. If you have general interest, we encourage you to explore a variety of meditation practices. And as is the case for many people, you might find meditation to be a health practice, like going to the gym, that helps strengthen your neural connections of focus and attention while reducing your stress and anxiety.

CONCENTRATIVE PRACTICES

Concentrative practices of meditation are common and often basic. You could do a quick practice right now by simply focusing on your breath, feeling yourself breathing in and breathing out for five or ten minutes. The goal is to concentrate on each breath and on what you feel during each of those breaths. By doing this for even a short period of time, you'll relax your brain and reduce your level of stress. Breath work meditations are among the most common and universal and also part of many spiritual traditions. The general idea is that breathing is a fundamental process of life, and focusing on the breath essentially gets you in touch with your basic life processes. Physiologically, by focusing on the slow rhythm of your breath, you activate the parasympathetic, or calming, part of your nervous system and cause an overall reduction in stress and anxiety.

Another simple concentrative practice is to focus your visual attention on a particular object and bring your full attention to its shape, movement, and color. For example, you can concentrate your visual energy on a candle flame or on objects that might especially have religious or spiritual meaning such as a cross, mandala, or other sacred symbol. This type of meditation for five to ten minutes is a way to reduce your stress in a short period of time.

We performed our own study on how the brain functions when focusing on specific religious or nonreligious symbols.[2] We showed people the following panel with depictions of a variety of symbols that had either religious or nonreligious meaning, as well as positive or negative emotional content as rated by the study participants themselves.

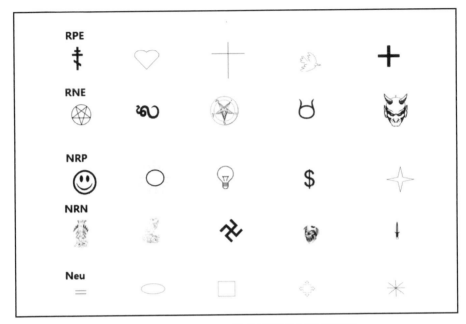

ILLUSTRATION COURTESY OF THE MARCUS INSTITUTE OF INTEGRATIVE HEALTH

We used functional MRI to demonstrate that the symbols with associated positive emotions, particularly if they were religious, were more likely to activate the primary visual system of the brain. This was an important finding because it showed that symbols have a profound impact on the brain before we are even aware of them. Thus, a simple meditation on a symbol that has great meaning to you can have profound effects on the way in which your brain functions.

One final variation on this notion of focusing on an object is to visualize that object in your mind. This can be somewhat more difficult because you have to cognitively maintain the image in your mind, but it can be a rewarding practice. The goal is to select a particular object that you like to focus on—a religious symbol, candle, mountain, ocean, or something else of meaning to you—bring your attention to it and visualize it in your mind, and then continue to concentrate on it. Our studies of Tibetan Buddhist meditation involved the participants' focusing intently on a visual sacred object. The results showed an increase in activation of the frontal lobes related to the focus and a decrease in activation in the parietal lobes associated with the sense of becoming one with the object.

Using images that you visualize in your mind during meditation is somewhat similar to practices referred to as *guided imagery*, a process by which you create certain visual images in your mind to help change the way your brain responds. For example, sometimes people talk about "going to their happy place." Thinking about a time at the beach or under a moonlit sky can be ways of using this visual imagery to relax your mind. A number of studies have also demonstrated that guided imagery techniques can be effective for reducing anxiety, depression, and stress. Many of these types of concentrative practices can be done on your own, but if you need additional support, it can be found online, through a phone app, or with local practitioners.

Another set of concentration techniques uses verbal objects. The most common type of verbal object is referred to as a mantra, which represents a specific sound or sounds that you repeat over and over. By concentrating on repeating them, you activate the language-producing areas of your brain in your frontal lobes which then have a regulating effect on the emotional centers of your brain and give a feeling of relaxation. And since you are performing a focusing task, the mantra also tends to augment function in the areas of the brain that can result in improved focus and attention. It may be particularly useful too for those who struggle with the concentration process, particularly those with attention-deficit hyperactivity disorder (ADHD). Well-known mantra-based programs include transcendental meditation (TM) in which you are given a unique mantra and the "OM" meditation in which you focus on the single mantra, "Om."

We have also studied the mantra-based practice Kirtan Kriya (please see pages 65–66). Our initial research on it showed that it increased activity in the frontal lobe by about 15 percent and similarly increased memory and attention by approximately 15 percent.[3] Although this meditation practice is considered to be one of the most basic forms in the Kundalini yoga tradition, it can be performed in a purely secularized manner with the goal of reducing stress and anxiety while augmenting attention, concentration, and memory.

Concentrative meditation techniques have generally been shown to reduce stress and anxiety. They are particularly good if you like to have something to focus on. Some of our patients have told us they prefer these practices because they get too distracted with extraneous thoughts during open monitoring approaches. Hence, if getting distracted is an issue for you, concentrative practices may be more useful because you do a particular task rather than simply keep your mind open. But as with every practice we describe, it is important to try it for a period of time to see if you enjoy doing it and you think it is providing a benefit. If at any time a meditation practice feels highly uncomfortable, frustrating, or unhelpful, we usually recommend moving on to a different one.

MINDFULNESS-BASED AWARENESS

In open monitoring or mindfulness-based awareness, or sometimes as awareness-based practices, the goal is not to focus your mind on any particular object or thought, but rather to allow various thoughts and experiences to enter your awareness, pay attention to them, and then let them go. Mindfulness meditation is one of the most common and certainly one of the most widely studied of these practices. We are big proponents of the formalized mindfulness-based stress reduction (MBSR) program. Our team at the Marcus Institute runs one of the largest mindfulness programs in the country in which we teach mindfulness techniques to both our patients and health professionals. In mindfulness, you engage a nonjudgmental awareness of whatever thoughts, feelings, or experiences enter into your mind. By being nonjudgmental, you keep from running away with your thoughts and are better able to self-regulate your emotional responses.

The early studies of mindfulness, as well as more recent ones, have demonstrated its effectiveness in people with high perceived stress. And for those with anxiety disorders or primary depression, it has been found to offer significant and persistent improvements in their symptoms.[4] One of the advantages of mindfulness is that the program itself has been well designed, well studied, well described, and well taught in a uniform way for a wide range of people. Thus, a mindfulness program in New York or Iowa will have a great deal of similarity. This codification of the practice has also made it easy for researchers to study using scientific methods.

The program is applicable whether you are struggling with your own illness, trying to navigate a pandemic, or feeling that the stresses of work and home are getting the best of you. For example, a patient recovering from colon cancer who gets a twinge of pain in her abdomen might suddenly begin to worry that her cancer has returned and she will have to go through difficult surgery and therapy, even though testing confirms that she is okay. A mindfulness program would ask her to stop that thought process at the beginning and simply accept the pain as an experience without going any further in trying to interpret it or worry about it, unless of course she really needs to. Mindfulness recognizes that anxiety can breed more anxiety. You may begin to feel nervous about something, and then become more nervous just from worrying about it. Again, mindfulness helps cut off this process where it begins. Another example is a busy executive who is starting to feel more fatigued and less productive because the stresses of life have become all-consuming. In this case, mindfulness practices would help create a space from the stressors and thereby facilitate her more adaptive and healthful coping.

A brain scan study of about thirty long-term mindfulness practitioners with over nine thousand hours of practice each and thirty people who went through just a standard eight-week mindfulness program showed that both groups had less reactivity in the amygdala—the fear and anxiety center in the brain—to overall emotional stimuli. Interestingly, both groups had the same reduction in reactivity to negative emotional stimuli, which implies that relatively short courses of mindfulness meditation can be effective in changing how the brain operates. However, longer-term practice, especially in an intense form, can change the brain even more, as evidenced by thicker frontal lobes in the long-term meditators compared to the beginners. The research clearly shows a training response, but in contrast to training to become a concert pianist or to perform open heart surgery, you might not require hours and hours before seeing positive results.

Thus, mindfulness can be a highly useful and successful mediation approach, especially if the full MBSR program is used. It certainly is an approach that has helped many in navigating the stressors in life. But mindfulness is not for everyone. Some people have difficulty allowing their awareness to just sit there and become too distracted to be able to perform the practice. Others have found that the practice is not consistent with their religious or spiritual beliefs, even though being a more mindful religious person can frequently augment their religious or spiritual beliefs. For example, you might enjoy going to a meeting of your religious practice more because you are able to experience the service, music, and rituals more intensely. This is true of virtually every other domain of life as well. Also, because of the successes of mindfulness, it is being incorporated into more standard approaches for psychological treatments. Hence, cognitive behavioral therapy has been enhanced with mindfulness in a way that builds on primary processes that help people overcome stressful situations, anxiety, and depression.

MOVING MEDITATIONS

Moving meditations can be particularly fun and useful for those who prefer to be in motion. If you just do not like sitting still for prolonged periods of time, you might find practices that involve walking or other body movements to be a more effective approach to help you reduce your stress and improve your brain function. Two of the most common types of moving meditation are yoga and tai chi. Yoga derives from the Hindu tradition and is a way to prime the body for meditative and spiritual experiences, though in our popular culture, yoga programs have typically been secularized so that little of the Hindu tradition is engaged. In this regard, yoga becomes more of a stretching exercise, yet still can be relaxing and therapeutic to the brain.

We performed an early study looking at the brain during yoga meditation and found that it provides similar effects as other types of meditation practices. In particular, yoga meditation enhanced frontal lobe function and reduced emotional reactivity.[5] You can see evidence of this in the brain imaging figures titled Yoga and the Brain in the color photography section. Hundreds of other studies have explored the effects of yoga meditation, and yoga in general, on mental health factors. Overall, yoga practices have been shown to be effective at reducing stress, anxiety, and depression.[6] These practices may also have benefits for various health concerns such as musculoskeletal conditions or asthma because of the focus on moving the body and increasing the breath. And for people with severe health conditions who are unable to participate in many yoga poses, programs such as Iyengar yoga can offer more support by using including pillow, chairs, and other aids. Importantly, if you are ever doing a yoga program and find it to be physically uncomfortable or painful, it is important to stop and modify the practice until it becomes comfortable. And if this is not possible, you may need to consider other types of practices.

Tai chi involves making motions with both your arms and legs as part of an overall meditative program. By slowly moving your arms and legs in a cyclical and rhythmic manner, you can achieve a state of deep relaxation. It can also be fun to do. Although there are not a large number of studies looking into tai chi and mental health, those that do exist have generally shown it to be beneficial along the same lines as yoga and other like-minded practices.[7]

While there are many other moving meditations, we close this section by addressing the most basic of all: meditating while walking. Taking a walk outdoors, even in the city, or as crazy as it might sound, around your office building, can be done as a meditative practice. The goal is to pay attention to everything going on around you while you are walking. Take in the moment, and reflect on what you are seeing, hearing, smelling, and touching. Notice as many details as possible using those four senses. Are there new plants you didn't notice before? What types of sounds do you hear: birds, traffic, people? How does the air smell? Are there things you can touch, like a flower, to feel more connected to the moment? Walking itself is well known to improve cardiovascular health as well as psychological health. Thus, we highly recommend walking meditation as a simple practice that can help you optimize your brain function and can be done in minutes.

SELECTING THE RIGHT MEDITATION FOR YOU

Although we have discussed a number of excellent meditation-based programs, an important question we always get from our patients and colleagues alike is how to figure out the right meditation for them. You can never know for sure which will work best for you until you try some out. But we offer several recommendations to help you in that process.

The first question to ask yourself is, *What is the goal of my meditation practice?* Are you planning on doing meditation to reduce stress, enhance cognition, or find spiritual meaning? Depending on your answer, you can already consider or reject certain types of meditation. Certainly, if your goal is something spiritual, you might want to move away from the secularized practices and explore those associated with various religious or sacred traditions.

The next question is, *Do I generally like to move around, or would I rather sit still?* If you are comfortable with sitting still, a number of practices satisfy that requirement. And if you prefer to move around, consider options such as yoga or tai chi.

Once you have answered these basics, you can then consider whether to start with practices that are well developed, well studied, and popular. While it certainly does not mean that these practices will necessarily be right for you, they obviously are right for many people and have a fair amount of data supporting them. If this is the direction you lean toward, practices like mindfulness and yoga are generally good starting points.

It is particularly important to do your homework by looking up the practice or, better yet, talking to the teacher who will be guiding you through it. Ask about the nature of the practice. Make sure that the approach is consistent with your own ideas, goals, and beliefs. If you sense that a particular teacher is going to put you under too much duress while doing the meditation practice, that one is probably not right for you. If you get a good feeling from a particular teacher that the practice will be something you can enjoy, engage in fully, and benefit from, that is certainly a practice worth giving a try. But in the end, give whatever practice you choose a reasonable try and see how you feel about it. You'll need at least a month or two to be able to determine how well it is working for you in terms of achieving your goals. You can always enhance your practice too with some of the other approaches we've mentioned. For example, if you choose to do transcendental meditation, you can also layer that with some walking meditations. Like everything else we've mentioned, the more you reinforce these meditative circuits in your brain, and the more diversity you add to those reinforcements, the better the outcome.

Chapter 13
SPECIAL TOOLS FOR BRAIN HEALTH

*Your brain never stops developing and changing. It's been doing it from
the time you were an embryo, and will keep on doing it all your life.*

—JAMES TREFIL, 1997

When it comes to weaving together the best brain possible, an intriguing part of the armamentarium comes in a variety of special tools that can help you activate or modulate your brain function. These tools, some high tech and some quite old, have been used in a number of ways for both keeping the brain healthy and helping with various cognitive issues. Many of these tools have not been studied to the extent modern medicine typically prefers before using them with the general population, but a number of research studies already show a variety of interesting and potentially beneficial effects. Of note, these tools are used by trained professionals, so for the most part, they are not do-it-yourself techniques. However, we want you to know about them because most are applied with tremendous success by our clinical and research team at the Marcus Institute of Integrative Health at Thomas Jefferson University. In general, these tools involve stimulating the brain directly or producing various patterns of activity in the brain through some type of feedback or focused approach that can help people change the way they think and feel. The tools we review here are hypnosis; biofeedback and neurofeedback; "energy psychology," which includes the Neuro Emotional Technique (NET); homeopathy; eye movement desensitization and reprocessing (EMDR); and transcranial magnetic stimulation (TMS).

HYPNOSIS

When most people think of hypnosis, they envision a stage performer making people act like chickens. But hypnosis has a long and complex history and has been used effectively for a variety of brain-related issues. It has been defined as "a state of consciousness involving focused attention and reduced peripheral awareness characterized by an enhanced capacity for response to suggestion."[1] The last part is how hypnosis typically offers therapeutic effects: it helps provide suggestions to people to alter problematic thoughts and behaviors.

The first use of hypnosis was by a French physician, Dr. Franz Anton Mesmer (1734–1815), frequently considered the father of hypnosis. You may also recognize his name as the root of a common word—*mesmerize*—which has come to be synonymous with the brain state achieved during hypnosis. Hypnosis as a therapeutic technique developed significantly over the nineteenth and twentieth centuries. An important aspect of it is a person's hypnotizability. Even Freud toyed with it a bit, though he ended up not incorporating it into the psychoanalytic method he became famous for. Hypnotizability is considered to be a trait that does not change much throughout the life of a person. However, it does seem to be affected by childhood experiences and is associated with creativity and the ability to utilize imagination and vivid imagery. There are even certain electroencephalogram (EEG) findings that can suggest how hypnotizable a person might be. The reason this trait is important is that it directly correlates with the potential success of hypnosis as a therapy. The more hypnotizable you are, the greater the magnitude of the therapeutic benefit you might expect.

Clinicians typically use an induction technique that incorporates focusing on the breath, relaxation, directing attention, and imagery to evoke memories of previous experiences that are similar to the hypnotic state. Interestingly, some researchers have induced hypnosis without the relaxation component, which suggests that even patients who are in stressful or unusual circumstances can be hypnotized. Although some describe hypnosis in terms of the process itself by using various cues and contexts, it clearly involves a complex interplay of genetics, brain structure, imagination, and patterns of neuronal networking. While there are not yet a lot of brain scan studies on this, hypnosis appears to be associated with activity changes in the frontal lobes.[2] This makes sense since the frontal lobes are involved in our ability to focus attention and modulate our emotions and beliefs. For instance, brain scan studies have shown that highly hypnotizable people tend to have more efficient frontal lobes, which enable them to enter into a so-called trance state more effectively and also to be more suggestible in that state.

Once a patient is under hypnosis, the clinician can offer restorative suggestions for a variety of concerns such as mood disorders and behavioral issues. A number of studies have demonstrated that hypnosis can be effective, especially for those dealing with specific types of harmful beliefs or habits. As an example, hypnosis has been used in patients facing substance abuse, particularly smoking, by helping them deal with related aspects, specifically cravings or other environmental stimuli. Often the therapy involves home practice using auto-hypnosis, plus audio recordings given to reinforce the work done in sessions with the clinician.

Although hypnosis is a difficult intervention to study using traditional means with placebo control groups, we have had some success in our clinic with patients who are struggling with smoking cessation, chronic pain, and other issues. The indications are that for the right person, it can be a tremendous tool in the overall treatment of their brain and body health.

BIOFEEDBACK

Biofeedback also has a long history with early roots dating back to the nineteenth century with more formal clinical applications having been developed over fifty years ago. The basic approach is to use certain physiological measures, such as heart rate or muscle contractions, that are typically handled by the brain automatically—meaning they occur without us thinking about them—and help bring them under some degree of voluntary control. This involves equipment that gives real-time feedback on what is going on physiologically. For example, if your goal is to lower your heart rate, the therapist will give you techniques, such as ones to relax your breathing, while a heart monitor shows how well you drive your heart rate to lower levels. And if you start to think of something that makes you anxious, say your taxes, they will see in real time how your heart rate goes up. For this reason, we are big proponents of using biofeedback in our full-day executive health program. As part of our head-to-toe assessments, our patients meet with our biofeedback therapist to learn which stressors affect their physiology in negative ways, and then we help empower them with tools to dampen or reverse those biological responses.

The mechanism behind biofeedback most likely involves some degree of control over the autonomic nervous system. This makes sense because the higher parts of the brain, such as the frontal lobe, can be used to concentrate and regulate emotional responses and, in turn, body responses. The frontal lobe connects through central structures such as the thalamus and hypothalamus, which then regulate the autonomic nervous system. But the brain can also regulate other physiological processes as well. Biofeedback programs can be set up to regulate skin conduction, respiration, and even electrical activity in the brain itself. For example, we have helped many patients with chronic headaches learn to better control their skin temperature.

For brain activity, by watching their electroencephalogram (EEG), our patients can observe their different brain wave patterns and over time modify them to be in more favorable brain wave states. This approach of using the brain to regulate itself is called *neurofeedback*. In the context of brain waves, if you want to be more relaxed, you might train your brain to fill up with relaxing alpha waves. Once you have gotten used to what that feels like, you will be able to elicit that sensation even without the help of an EEG. The usual goal of neurofeedback is to help reprogram the brain to reduce stress and anxiety and improve focus and attention. As you can imagine, neurofeedback programs have gotten rather sophisticated. Some of the activities can feel like playing games or engaging in something enjoyable like learning to modulate the perception of a sunrise so that it points the brain's electrical activity in a desirable direction. While data on clinical outcomes are limited, some studies show it can be effective.

Newer approaches to neurofeedback, particularly in the research realm, include using functional magnetic resonance imaging (fMRI) to observe changes in the brain's activity, as measured by blood flow, on a moment-to-moment basis.[3] Much like an EEG, you can use this form of neurofeedback to modify the amount of activity in different parts of your brain. For example, if certain parts are imbalanced, either high or low in their activity, neurofeedback can be a way to help rebalance the brain. Since fMRI is still relatively new, and certainly much more expensive than EEG, this type of MRI-based neurofeedback is still being developed. But the initial research is promising.

NEURO EMOTIONAL TECHNIQUE

Neuro Emotional Technique (NET) is a novel mind-body intervention that we use a lot at the Marcus Institute in our clinical and research programs. Our early research on effectiveness has been quite impressive, which is why we also teach the intervention in our academic programs for health care providers.

NET is sometimes classified as an energy psychology tool because it incorporates acupressure points and the acupuncture meridian system, along with muscle biofeedback, autonomic nervous system modulation, and psychological principles of learning theory, cognitive behavioral therapy, and others. Our groundbreaking research on NET has shown through brain scans that the functional activity of the brain dramatically changed after the technique was applied, particularly when patients were coping with stressful events.[4] One of the results we were most impressed by in these studies was the dramatic difference in how the brain functioned, which corresponded to patients' subjective reports that they felt improvements after just a few sessions. Dan's recent book, *Tapestry of Health*, provides a deeper discussion of this technique with case examples and color images showing some of the changes in brain function that resulted.

HOMEOPATHY

Another modality that focuses on energy is homeopathy. In contrast to most other approaches, homeopathy takes a different perspective on how the brain and body work. Its basis centers primarily on the notion of using prepared substances that produce various symptoms associated with illnesses. These "similars," as they are called, are then diluted thousands or even millions of times. While the original molecules essentially are no longer in the dilution, it is believed that the effects are still incorporated through a kind of energetic signature. The theory is that giving someone a homeopathic remedy of that something in its diluted state would produce symptoms similar to the ones they are fighting and may help to improve those very symptoms.

Homeopathy was developed by a German physician, Samuel Hahnemann, and advanced in 1810 through his publication of *Organon of Rational Medicine* (in German: *Organon der rationellen Heilkunst*). He tested hundreds of animal, plant, mineral, and synthetic compounds with the goal of determining which ones and their dilutions had clinical effects. According to his theory, the more diluted a compound is, the stronger is its affect. He developed all of this into a compendium titled the *Materia Medica*.

Perhaps the greatest concern with homeopathy is that it has no clear relationship to how we understand physiological processes in the brain and body and how best to manage them. However, a number of studies have shown that homeopathic remedies can be beneficial, especially in a variety of brain-related disorders such as insomnia, depression, and anxiety.[5] In fact, a well-known article by Klaus Linde[6] and colleagues looked at all of the available literature and found that homeopathy seemed to work in a variety of conditions, including allergies and asthma, gastrointestinal problems, musculoskeletal issues, headaches, and premenstrual syndrome. And many interventions such as NET use homeopathy as a supportive tool.

Overall, homeopathy has a long tradition and history, and there are numerous types of data suggesting possible efficacy, albeit through a poorly understood mechanism of action. These remedies are generally safe; however, not all studies are positive, and most would agree that homeopathy needs much more research for it to be recommended as a primary treatment modality.

EYE MOVEMENT DESENSITIZATION AND REPROCESSING

A relatively new approach to help with specific psychological concerns such as post-traumatic stress disorder (PTSD) is eye movement desensitization and reprocessing (EMDR). This treatment involves inducing a series of rapid and rhythmic eye movements, and sometimes sounds, with the goal of reducing anxiety and helping with cognitive restructuring. Here's an example of the process: A patient typically brings to the forefront of his mind some type of negative memory or emotion associated with a trauma. He then engages in these rapid eye movements with the goal of reducing or eliminating their strong negative emotional reaction and replacing it with a more positive one. EMDR appears to work relatively quickly and as well as, if not better than, other approaches to help with PTSD. In fact, a substantial number of studies have shown the effectiveness of EMDR in different patient populations, including those with depression and anxiety.[7]

Although the mechanism is not fully understood yet, some interesting evidence supports the idea that EMDR works on the circuitry connecting the default mode network and the cerebellum. The cerebellum was also a factor in our studies showing the effectiveness of NET. Overall, EMDR appears to be a way to help balance the brain's responses to negative stimuli for a number of conditions, including PTSD. The technique might also be useful for those with mood disorders such as depression, but more data are needed.

TRANSCRANIAL MAGNETIC STIMULATION

Transcranial magnetic stimulation (TMS) is a newer technology approved by the Food and Drug Administration (FDA) as an adjunct treatment for depression and obsessive-compulsive disorder. This intervention is generally done under the close supervision of a physician specializing in psychiatry. TMS uses magnetic fields and takes advantage of the relationship between electricity and magnetism. By using certain types of magnetic fields, the electrical behavior of nerve cells can be affected in ways that alter their activity either higher or lower. The goal is to try to balance the brain's nerve cells more effectively by reducing areas that are overactive and raising areas that are underactive. By determining which areas are acting abnormally, the therapy can focus on just those regions and minimize the effects on other regions. Another advantage is that no drugs are involved with TMS, so the risk of side effects and drug interactions is greatly reduced.

A newly evolving device, transcranial direct current stimulation (tDCS), bypasses the magnetic fields and uses electricity to directly stimulate the nerve cells in different parts of the brain. It is important to note that this type of device is still in the exploratory stages and is not approved by the FDA. The roots of this approach go back as early as 1801, when Giovanni Aldini started a study in which he apparently successfully used direct current stimulation to improve the mood of some of his patients with melancholy. Preliminary studies of modern tDCS suggest it might also be a useful adjunctive treatment for anxiety and depression.[8] By stimulating the prefrontal cortex, tDCS may even reduce substance craving in patients with addiction.[9] More research is needed, but since this may be an up-and-coming modality, we want to relay to you what is known to date.

CHOOSING SPECIAL TOOLS TO HELP YOUR BRAIN

In the end, the choice of which special tools you might want to use to help your brain depends on the specific issues you are trying to manage. Most important, each of these tools requires expert guidance, so talk with your physician or therapist to assess which might be best for you. Also remember that these methods are primarily treatments for those managing some type of psychological or brain disorder rather than for those wanting to optimize their brain function.

PART THREE

Dealing with Brain Problems

Chapter 14

ANXIETY

*Adrenaline, dopamine, oxytocin. The drugstore of the brain
does not ask if you have a prescription.*

—JERRY SEINFELD, 2020

Anxiety disorders affect about 40 million American adults each year, but everyone who has ever walked on this planet experiences anxiety, defined as "the apprehensive anticipation of future danger or misfortune accompanied by a feeling of dysphoria or somatic symptoms of tension. The focus of anticipated danger may be internal or external."[1] This kind of reaction is important for your overall survival because it helps you avoid danger. But anxiety, while stimulating your autonomic nervous system in the short run, ends up reducing its reactivity in the long run. Too much anxiety is characterized by excessive and persistent nervousness, worrying, fear, irritability, and sleep disturbances. And since the brain and body are intimately connected, a lot of physical symptoms can accompany anxiety, such as sweating, palpitations, chest pain, headaches, difficulty concentrating, and muscle tension. Excessive anxiety affects almost every system of the body: digestive, cardiovascular, and even immune function.

While it's normal to feel anxious from time to time, there are a variety of specific anxiety disorders, including generalized anxiety disorder, the most common type; anxiety disorder due to a medical condition such as cancer; substance-induced anxiety disorder; panic attacks that are acute episodes of intense anxiety; agoraphobia, which is a fear of going out and being with other people; phobias, which are irrational fears and anxieties about specific things like spiders or heights; obsessive-compulsive disorder (OCD), which is related to specific behaviors associated with anxiety symptoms; and post-traumatic stress disorder (PTSD), which is when intense anxiety is associated with one or more specific life-threatening events such as being in combat, a car accident, or a violent attack.

While our focus here is nonpathological anxiety, many of the approaches we discuss can be used as part of an overall plan for those who have a true anxiety disorder or even for proactively protecting against the development of PTSD. After all, what we all have in common is trying to find ways to navigate our anxieties and traumas so that we can function and feel better, healthier, and more whole. This is where our entire discussion about becoming a good brain weaver through the tools and approach of integrative medicine comes into play. When patients need medication for anxiety or anything else, we prescribe it. But as part of our integrative model of care, we also use other modalities whenever possible, as well as innovative wellness strategies to add value to a medical treatment plan. And the stronger your brain is to begin with, the more it will be responsive to solutions for various challenges and traumas in life.[2]

Our goal is to treat all aspects of a person by addressing their four dimensions—the biological, psychological, social, and spiritual—because it is essential that these four work in harmony for optimal health and well-being.

THE BRAIN AND ANXIETY

As we briefly review some of the underlying pathophysiology of anxiety in the brain and nervous system, it is important to keep in mind from earlier chapters the discussions on the downstream effects of this biology on your organs, inflammation levels, and immune system. A physiological way of thinking about excessive anxiety is that it is a stress response on overdrive. Basically, the stress response is most often triggered when survival of the organism is perceived to be threatened, whether or not it actually is. When this happens, the activation of the sympathetic/arousal nervous system results in increased heart rate, blood pressure, and respiratory rate. Brain scan studies also show intense activation of alerting areas of the brain such as the hypothalamus and amygdala, although the network of structures involved in this stress response is much more complicated and may also incorporate many other brain structures.[3] What follows in the body is the release of the main stress hormone, cortisol, along with adrenaline, which engages the body to be on alert.

For someone who has too much anxiety or even an anxiety disorder, there is usually a dysregulation of the stress response, as well as substantial changes in a number of neurotransmitter systems, the chemicals that the nervous system uses to communicate with the rest of the body.[4] We have previously mentioned gamma-aminobutyric acid (GABA) as being the primary inhibitory central nervous system neurotransmitter, but it appears to be markedly decreased in people with panic disorders.[5] This implies that individuals are not able to modulate their fear or stress response effectively, which causes them increased and sustained anxiety. In addition, other neurotransmitters such as epinephrine and norepinephrine are released in the brain and body and activate many more processes that can lead to a faster heart rate and higher blood pressure, for example.

Given these brain findings, we consider a variety of integrative medicine approaches for the management of nonpathological anxiety based on the following four tiers. The first brings together diet, nutrition, and exercise. Mind-body therapies and psychotherapeutic approaches make up the second tier. The third tier includes supplements and herbal remedies, and medications, when necessary, represents the fourth tier.

DIETARY INFLUENCES ON ANXIETY

In chapter 2 on diet and nutrition, as well as chapter 10 on stress, we emphasized the importance of a healthy diet on weaving together a healthy brain. We also discussed how foods that have a lot of processed ingredients, high carbohydrate loads, and bad fats end up causing a great deal of inflammation in your brain and body. This inflammation can trigger the same molecules involved in your stress or anxiety response. For example, an early study in Australia found that a traditional dietary pattern characterized by vegetables, fruit, meat, fish, and whole grains was associated with lower odds for having depression and anxiety disorders. This association held even after adjusting for age, socioeconomic status, education, and lifestyle behaviors. Other studies have also shown a healthy diet consisting of high-protein and high-plant-based foods is associated with a much more balanced brain state and less anxiety. At the opposite end of the spectrum, a Western diet consisting of processed and fried foods, refined grains, added sugars, and beer was associated with much higher anxiety scores.[6] In a follow-up study, this same research team showed that the "standard American diet," for which they cleverly developed the acronym "SAD," full of processed meats, pizza, salty snacks, sweets, soft drinks, French fries, margaritas, cake, and ice cream, yielded a significantly higher likelihood of having anxiety symptoms.[7]

Foods that have direct toxic biochemical effects—for instance, ones that cause increased inflammation—may also have direct deleterious physiological effects including impaired cardiovascular function. For example, if you consume something with a high glycemic index—a high sugar content that sharply elevates blood sugar levels—such as a can of soda on an empty stomach, you initially get a high amount of sugar coursing through your bloodstream. To compensate, your body releases insulin to drive your sugar levels back down. But your body may overshoot on the insulin in overcompensating for the sugar surge, resulting in the familiar hypoglycemic crash, leaving you feeling lethargic and with cloudy thinking. Worse still, your body does not like to be hypoglycemic and gets stressed out, which means it then releases all that cortisol, epinephrine, and norepinephrine.[8] While this whole response helps restore your glucose levels toward normal, it also induces your fight-or-flight response, which can manifest in anxiety, palpitations, and irritability and affect white blood cells by releasing inflammatory chemicals and impairing your immunity. The best way to combat this is to eat foods that are high in protein and avoid simple carbohydrates like white bread, white rice, refined pasta, and sugary foods so you don't have wild swings in your blood sugar and mood.

In chapter 3 on the gut-brain connection, we described how the types of bacteria in your gut are directly connected to your brain functions. Similarly, there is a strong relationship between gut bacteria and anxiety, for several reasons. One is that if there are abnormal amounts of bad bacteria in the gut, it results in chronic inflammation, which then triggers the immune system into action. In addition, increased inflammation in the body may be associated with increased anxiety symptoms. So it is important to maintain a good diet and consider ways to keep a healthy gut flora. Studies suggest that probiotics might be helpful in this regard, but there are no clear data with respect to anxiety itself.

Emerging research also has found that microbiota help modulate serotonin and GABA signaling in the brain and body.[9] This entire gut-brain relationship is probably much more intricate than we know. Bidirectional communication between the two is now recognized as likely playing a key role in a number of psychological conditions such as anxiety and depression. The important point here is that to help your anxiety, you must take good care of your gut, and the best way to do that is to eat a plant-based, protein-based diet and to minimize processed foods, refined sugars, and starches.

There are some additional, perhaps obvious, recommendations to consider from a dietary standpoint when it comes to managing anxiety. Specifically, stop eating foods that have a stimulatory effect, such as caffeine. Anything that stimulates your nervous system is also going to increase your chances of feeling anxious because they excite your brain and increase your heart rate, so quitting or greatly eliminating caffeine, alcohol, and smoking are all going to help you manage your anxiety symptoms.[10] Another issue with these substances is that if you have been using them for some time, you might experience withdrawal symptoms, which can feel a lot like, you guessed it, anxiety.

EXERCISE

We have already sung the praises of regular physical activity as one of the best ways to manage anxiety and build your best brain. In fact, physical inactivity has been demonstrated to be a risk factor for the development of a variety of behavioral illnesses, including anxiety.[11] When you exercise, it is as if you use up most of your anxiety-producing hormones and afterward are more relaxed.

Physiologically it results in the release of endorphins, which produce relaxation, and serotonin, which improves mood. Exercise is a critical component of optimal brain health, especially when you feel anxious.

According to the American Psychiatric Association, current best practice guidelines for the treatment of anxiety disorders include regular physical activity such as walking for an hour or running twenty to thirty minutes at least four days a week. A recent meta-analysis looking at a large number of research studies found that exercise as a therapeutic intervention is as effective as psychotherapy, and almost as effective as medication, for the treatment of anxiety symptoms.[12]

MIND-BODY MODALITIES

We have discussed a variety of mind-body practices in previous chapters on meditation and spirituality, practices that generally are particularly good for helping with anxiety. By themselves, they are not likely to be a primary treatment for anxiety disorders. However, they can be wonderful adjunctive modalities to help with normal, everyday stressors or life-stopping panic attacks and anxiety disorders.

The Mindfulness-Based Stress Reduction program (MBSR), described earlier and one of the most studied meditation-based programs with over three hundred scientific articles published about it, has been shown to significantly reduce symptoms of stress and anxiety.[13] The basic MBSR program runs eight weeks and is highly standardized so that you can have a similar experience no matter where you take it as long as the instructor is certified in teaching the course. In mindfulness, the primary goal is to remain in the present moment using nonjudgmental awareness of your thoughts and feelings.

When Jon Kabat-Zinn developed the MBSR program and first tested it in 1992 on twenty-two patients with panic disorder or generalized anxiety disorder, he found the participants had a significant improvement in their anxiety and panic symptoms. The mechanism may also include an overall reduction in stress, as well as an important psychological change, by emphasizing a more neutral approach in the way people view their negative thoughts and stressors. This occurs because the program apparently increases activity in the frontal lobe, which then helps decrease activity in the amygdala. In addition, the practice alters serotonin and dopamine levels, which contributes to more positive emotions.[14]

Guided imagery approaches can also help reduce anxiety. The proverbial "going to your happy place" by imagining a beach or peaceful mountainside can help take your mind off your worries and relax your brain and body. Guided imagery approaches can also be more specific. One study showed that patients who visualized making a successful speech were able to reduce their stress when they actually gave the speech in person. Basically, if you visualize positive things happening to you, you will feel less stress and likely be more effective in your tasks.

Yoga, the mind-body practice involving stretches, breath control, movement, and meditation, has a lot of research, including a larger systematic review of eight studies, showing that it significantly reduces anxiety symptoms in a variety of populations, even in children.

Tai chi and qi gong are two other forms of moving meditations, and ones that have been practiced in China for centuries though they are relative newcomers in the United States. They have been shown to significantly reduce anxiety and cortisol levels. In fact, a systematic review of sixty-eight studies reported that tai chi significantly reduced anxiety symptoms, especially in students of higher education.[15]

Music and, more specifically, music therapy have generally been shown to be effective for reducing anxiety. Music therapy is essentially a controlled form of listening to music applied in a number of settings, such as a doctor's office or a surgical suite, with the specific goal of improving a psychological or physical state.[16] The results of these studies show that playing peaceful music can help calm both patients and health care providers and lead to better overall medical outcomes. Not only does music itself support the slow rhythms of your body, which leads to relaxation, it can also screen out many unpleasant and unfamiliar sounds that frequently increase anxiety.[17]

As with everything else we have emphasized in this book, it is most important to find music that works specifically for you. This can require several sessions with a music therapist to determine which style of music and volume, tone, and tempo are most beneficial for inducing in you a feeling of relaxation and decreased anxiety. Or you can try this on your own to see which pieces in your music library can be put together into an antianxiety playlist. Find songs that relax you, uplift you, and help take your mind away from life's stressors. Doing this for even several minutes at a time, several times per day, can have a marked effect on reducing your anxiety.

Art therapy is a creative process that can help you express your feelings more effectively and subsequently reduce your anxiety. The artwork itself can be any modality of interest to you—for example, drawing, creating collages, or molding pottery. A number of studies have demonstrated a resulting reduction in anxiety and depressive symptoms in various patient populations, including those with cancer or stroke.[18] Thus, if doing art is something you particularly like, it can be a wonderful emotional outlet and highly useful for reducing your anxiety symptoms.

Aromatherapy uses essential oils from plants to release relaxing fragrances with the goal of reducing stress and anxiety. Interestingly, a number of studies exploring aromatherapy in specific medical environments, such as those where colonoscopies or surgeries are performed, did not show improvements in patient anxiety. However, many people find that pleasant aromas help them relax, and if you are one of those, you might consider getting some scented candles or oils for your home or workplace as a way to help you feel more comfortable.

Finally, massage therapy has been explored in specific patient populations, such as those with cancer or chronic pain, and has been found to reduce their anxiety. One study even showed that massage was helpful for reducing anxiety in hospital patients being treated for substance abuse and withdrawals from alcohol, cocaine, and opiates.[19]

What all of these studies of mind-body practices show is that these techniques are particularly useful in helping people cope with anxiety. Depending on the issues you face, how much anxiety you have, and which types of programs seem best suited to you and your life, try exploring them to find what works best for you.

SPIRITUALITY

When it comes to the relationship between spirituality and anxiety, growing evidence supports that spiritual practices and beliefs can be of great benefit. Of course, the impact of religious and spiritual activities on anxiety is probably multifactorial. Certainly, the social support alone can be a great factor in coping with significant life stressors.

Many of the prayer practices and other rituals can be considered a form of mind-body approach to alleviating stress and anxiety. For example, intensive prayer is similar to meditation and by itself can help lower your heart rate, blood pressure, and overall autonomic function so that you feel less stressed and anxious. Also, our study that looked at the effects of the rosary in Catholic patients with anxiety results showed that the patients who did the rosary were significantly better at reducing their anxiety than the control group, which simply received educational information about anxiety. The rosary has limitations in applying specifically to Catholics, yet virtually every tradition, religious or not, has rituals like the rosary that you can choose to perform as a way to help manage anxiety.

One final point about religious and spiritual beliefs is how they help us deal with the overarching human anxiety that we sometimes refer to as *ontological anxiety*. While people are usually anxious about specific things, there are also sovmetimes background anxieties about what the meaning of life is, how to behave morally, and what the whole universe is doing anyway. Although we do not focus on these big-picture anxieties very often, they can creep into our daily angsts as we struggle with various life issues such as helping a dying parent or deciding about ending a relationship. The classic midlife crisis can certainly apply here at a time when some people struggle to find purpose.

PSYCHOTHERAPEUTIC INTERVENTIONS

Psychotherapeutic approaches are widely recognized as appropriate nonpharmacological treatment for patients with anxiety disorders, and certainly they can be useful for people dealing with everyday anxiety as well. Cognitive behavioral therapy (CBT) takes a practical approach to personal problem solving by helping each patient change maladaptive patterns of thinking that can lead to increasing anxiety.[20] CBT works by combining psychoeducation, relaxation training, cognitive restructuring, and behavioral modification. The data show that approximately 50 to 65 percent of patients with anxiety disorders benefit from CBT.[21]

Since the MBSR program is highly effective for managing anxiety as well and since it seems to help with challenges like cognitive restructuring and relaxation training, some new approaches bring together mindfulness with CBT. Thus was born mindfulness-based cognitive therapy (MBCT). It has been documented to lessen anxiety and can also be a good approach if you want to embrace meditation as a fundamental part of your life too.[22]

Exposure therapy is another approach based on exposing patients in a systematic manner to their typical stressful or anxiety-provoking situations and stimuli.[23] This approach has also been called *systematic desensitization* because patients go step-by-step through their fear-related events and work toward reducing their stress response to each subsequent exposure. Over time, their anxiety levels can decrease.

Psychodynamic therapy focuses on core conflictual relationship themes and unconscious processes that affect a person's emotions, thoughts, and behaviors. By creating a deeper self-awareness and understanding of their own issues and mental processes, they can find ways to reduce their dysfunctional behaviors and relationships in order to reduce their overall anxiety. In fact, psychodynamic therapy has been shown to be as effective as CBT in patients with anxiety, and with beneficial effects lasting for at least one year.[24]

Rational emotive behavior therapy (REBT) is yet another therapeutic system that takes into account how a person's emotions, actions, and thoughts are interwoven. The theory is that early in life, we develop ineffectual or detrimental modes of managing various aspects of life. This therapy attempts to show the ways in which we inherently upset ourselves and then tries to help us retrain our behaviors by altering negative approaches and finding more effective ones that can lead to a happier, less anxious life.[25]

One reason we have provided this brief list and description of psychotherapeutic options, which are also generally applicable for depression, is that if you feel any of them is right for you, that some of the key concepts resonate with you, then you will look further into which might best help with soothing your own anxieties. For example, if you feel you have specific events that trigger anxiety, perhaps systematic desensitization would be better, or if you feel you are not handling your general approach to life as effectively as possible, perhaps REBT would be best. The point, at the risk of being repetitious, is to find the approach that works best for you. And it is most important to directly speak with any potential teacher, trainer, or therapist to find out what their strategy is and whether they feel like a good fit for you.

USE OF SUPPLEMENTS FOR ANXIETY

A wide variety of supplements have been explored for their potential use in patients with anxiety. Some supplements, such as vitamins and minerals, help to remedy nutritional deficiencies that may contribute to anxiety symptoms. Other supplements, such as natural molecules and botanicals, have a variety of compounds that can help reduce anxiety. We must stress, though, that when you take a supplement, even if it is "natural," it must be regarded as a drug in terms of whether it is effective, has side effects, and potentially interacts with other medications you might be taking. It is always important to discuss with your doctors any supplements or drugs you are taking so they can help ensure that the aids work as best as possible and don't cause problems.

Magnesium is important in many biochemical reactions and is involved in a wide range of physiological processes including the electrical properties and excitability of neurons. It is also a cofactor for more than three hundred different enzymes. Although foods such as nuts, whole grains, legumes, and green leafy vegetables contain a lot of magnesium, sometimes you might need a little extra. The ideal dosage of magnesium is 100 to 500 milligrams per day, with the primary side effect being loose stools. Among the different forms of magnesium that you can use, we typically recommend magnesium citrate since it is better absorbed and causes fewer side effects, but many supplements contain magnesium oxide because it has a low cost and a high concentration of elemental magnesium. One large double-blind study showed that magnesium in combination with an herbal formula significantly decreased mild to moderate anxiety when taken over a three-month period.[26]

While a variety of vitamins, including A, B, and D, taken individually or in a multivitamin, are involved in a number of cellular processes that can help your brain function more effectively overall, several studies have also found these nutrients to be beneficial specifically for reducing anxiety symptoms.

BOTANICALS

Several studies have shown that lavender oil (*Lavandula angustifolia*) can produce a calming, soothing response. In fact, one study of seventy-seven patients with generalized anxiety disorder did just as well with lavender oil as with benzodiazepine antianxiety medication. An even larger trial showed that lavender oil applied at 80 milligrams per day for ten weeks significantly lowered anxiety compared to those receiving a placebo.[27]

Lemon balm (*Melissa officinalis*) also has calming, soothing, antispasmodic, and anxiolytic effects.[28] While there are no large-scale trials in people with anxiety disorders, several small studies have shown that it increases feelings of calmness in healthy participants.[29]

Passionflower (*Passiflora incarnata*) is another botanical that has been shown to reduce anxiety symptoms. In one study in patients with generalized anxiety disorder, passionflower extract worked as well as the antianxiety medication oxazepam and produced fewer side effects.

Valerian (*Valeriana officinalis*) has long been used to help with sleeping better because of its calming, anxiolytic, and antispasmodic effects. It is typically given in doses of 300 milligrams, three times per day. Similar to the other compounds we have considered, one valerian study showed that it was as good as an antianxiety medication. But it is important to emphasize that valerian takes several weeks to kick in so it is not useful in an acute situation such as a panic attack.

Chamomile (*Matricaria chamomilla*) has calming effects and helps reduce anxiety when given at doses of approximately 200 to 220 milligrams per day. Yet one study of 179 patients with generalized anxiety disorder who took 500 milligrams of chamomile, three times per day, found significant reductions in anxiety symptoms in these patients with minimal side effects compared to a placebo.[30]

Kava kava (*Piper methysticum*) has antianxiety effects that seem to be associated with its constituents kavalactones, which directly alter how a neuron fires and may also be involved with GABA receptors that inhibit or turn off neurons. One result of these mechanisms is they reduce neuronal firings and anxiety symptoms. In fact a large meta-analysis found kava kava to be effective in regulating anxiety levels.[31] Standardized preparations typically contain 100 to 200 milligrams of kavalactones per day. But it can cause liver damage, so it is important to have your liver functions checked regularly by your doctor if you want to take kava kava.

MEDICAL TREATMENT

A number of drugs are also considered to be beneficial for managing anxiety and anxiety disorders, and we end this chapter with them to round out our integrative approach. We do not typically recommend these medications unless the patient has a more severe case or other treatment options have not worked. While the prescriptions help well with anxiety, they also have a number of side effects and, perhaps most problematic, can become addicting.

Interestingly, the first-line medical therapy for anxiety issues are not antianxiety medications but antidepressants. The most common ones are selective serotonin reuptake inhibitors (SSRIs) such as Prozac, Zoloft, or Celexa. These are recommended first since they have a lower likelihood of producing drowsiness and addiction. But they do not have an immediate effect, and it can be weeks before a change in the patient's baseline anxiety is seen. And like all other drugs, they have side effects. The ones common for SSRIs are gastrointestinal discomfort, reduced sexual interest and delayed orgasm, and weight gain. Sexual dysfunction, in particular, leads many patients to discontinue this treatment. A related class of medications, serotonin and norepinephrine reuptake inhibitors (SNRIs), affects both serotonin and norepinephrine (remember these are among the main stress neurotransmitters). These medications, including venlafaxine and duloxetine, or those prescribed by brand names including Effexor and Cymbalta, can be highly effective for treating anxiety disorders through the combined approach of changing the serotonin and norepinephrine neurotransmitter systems.

Benzodiazepines are well-known antianxiety medications that work by increasing activity at the GABA receptors, which subsequently turns off neurons that are overactive and causing anxiousness. A few common benzodiazepines are Xanax, Klonopin, Ativan, and Valium. Their main advantage over other medications is they work quickly, some of them even within minutes, but they can be highly addictive and the faster-acting ones are the most addictive. The other major side effects are drowsiness and diminished cognition, which can lead to accidents or injuries while driving or at work, sleep disturbances, and other psychiatric issues.

An interesting alternative, especially for performance-related anxiety such as public speaking, is the use of a beta-blocker. Common beta-blockers, such as propranolol and atenolol, or those prescribed by brand names including Inderal and Tenormin, are frequently used in cardiac patients to reduce their heart rate and blood pressure. The physical manifestations of anxiety in your body, like increased heart rate and blood pressure, are caused by the activation of the sympathetic arm of your autonomic nervous system. In the case of situational or performance anxiety, a cyclical process occurs whereby the anxious response in your brain leads to a heightened sympathetic nervous system that produces physical symptoms such as shortness of breath or flushing skin, perpetuates your anxiety, and keeps the response loop going around and around. Since these types of drugs generally do not cause drowsiness, interfere with cognition, or have significant side effects, they are generally the best medications for coping with stressful performance situations. There is even some evidence from a systematic review that found the beta-blocker propranolol can work just as well as the benzodiazepines to help manage panic disorders. But it is really designed for acute situations rather than for long-term treatment. The other thing to watch out for is that since propranolol lowers heart rate and blood pressure, if it has too strong of an effect, the patient can become lightheaded or even pass out.

Newer pharmacological approaches for the treatment of anxiety disorders are continually being explored. One interesting path is a return to old drugs that have psychedelic effects, such as psilocybin and LSD. A few early studies have shown potential therapeutic promise that they help in reducing anxiety.[32] This is an important area to pay attention to, and a number of new and ongoing studies are trying to figure out who responds well to these psychedelics and who does not.

Overall, a number of potentially effective integrative approaches help with anxiety symptoms and anxiety disorders. But remember that anxiety is a natural emotional and physiological response that triggers survivalist impulses for those in potentially dangerous situations. When experienced in appropriate amounts, it is adaptive, but if it becomes too much or for too long, it can impair your brain function and interfere with your life. Maintaining a healthy brain should help you keep your natural anxiety at healthy levels too.

Chapter 15

WEAVING TOGETHER
AN ELEVATED MOOD

The wound is the place where the Light enters you.

—RUMI, CIRCA 1258

*D*epressed, *low energy*, and *bad mood* are all terms used generically to describe a state of being that each of us feels from time to time. However, as with anxiety, when this state occurs too often, it can inhibit the brain's optimal functioning and exacerbate other issues.

Our focus for this chapter is on nonpathological depression that does not require psychiatric or medical care. In cases of significant depression, it is important to see a psychiatrist for appropriate treatment—for example, to get a prescription for medication—and then be carefully monitored by that physician. True mood disorders are a group of brain issues that include major depressive disorder, seasonal affective disorder, dysthymia, and bipolar disorder. While they require management from a trained mental health professional, we believe that our integrative approaches can also give added value to conventional care.

From our perspective, all mood issues, from grumpiness because stress has gotten out of control to genetically based bipolar disorder, are problems with the brain's functioning versus the ambiguous categorization of "mental illnesses." We believe this distinction is important for two reasons. First, we want to get away from the long-standing stigma associated with these conditions. They are common and important, and they need to be addressed aggressively. Calling them brain function problems makes them more tangible and biological. Second, because they have a biological and psychological side, we must consider a wide variety of approaches that can help. The goal is to try to restore the brain's functioning using our bio-psycho-social-spiritual model.

Addressing depression in general is challenging, and like so many other brain concerns, people can get caught up in a vicious cycle. For example, those with depression frequently don't eat well, don't sleep well, and don't engage with the world well. Poor diet, poor sleep, and poor social support make their depressive symptoms worse. It can be quite frustrating, but it is essential to find the right path out of that cycle. For our own patients, sometimes we start with their sleep, other times their diet. Like everything else we do in integrative medicine, the approach is tailored to the unique needs of the individual. What follows is a discussion of a variety of integrative approaches to help you bolster your mood and live with healthier brain functions. Again, we emphasize that anyone with a true mood disorder needs to be under the care of a trained clinician for guidance through the process.

DEPRESSION AND THE BRAIN

On one level, the relationship between depression and the brain is quite simple. But as with everything else regarding the brain, there are a lot of subtleties and complexities to contend with as well. The simple explanation for depression is that the brain's overall function is also depressed. This intuitively makes sense since depression is associated with reduced mood, reduced cognition, and reduced energy; it also makes sense, then, that the brain itself will have reduced activity. The very first paper Andy published documented how depression, especially in older individuals, is associated with an overall decrease in metabolic activity in the brain.[1] The decreased activity was even worse in depressed patients than it was in patients with Alzheimer's disease. This is quite remarkable since Alzheimer's is a neurodegenerative disorder that destroys neurons, whereas depression is a more functional issue in which neurons are just not working well. The data suggest that they are *really* not working well. With this simplified perspective, the obvious approach to depression is to try to increase activity in the brain.

Depression itself, though, is not simple. There are people who have different patterns of brain activity, including some who have higher metabolism in certain brain regions. The result is a brain that is imbalanced, and that is what causes the depressive symptoms. So, yes, we partly have to increase brain activity, but we have to do it carefully to help rebalance the brain in the process.

Underlying your brain's metabolic activity are neurotransmitters that regulate communication between different parts. We'll explain this a little further. Antidepressants are typically medications that affect the amount of serotonin, and sometimes dopamine or norepinephrine levels, in the brain. Serotonin appears to be the major mover when it comes to depression. When serotonin activity is low, the brain's activity is low. And if serotonin function can be augmented, the symptoms of depression can be slowly relieved. Again, this certainly is not a one-size-fits-all solution. Because of the brain balancing issue, sometimes just increasing the serotonin levels can make people feel worse. The goal is to find a way of individualizing therapy based on each person's unique depressive symptoms and constitution, and on more precise diagnostic tests such as their brain scans, to figure out what is going on in their brain. With a comprehensive amount of information, we can then help each patient find the best path out of depression.

DIET, NUTRITION, AND EXERCISE

As with all brain imbalances, diet is important in the treatment of a low mood. That means that adopting a brain-healthy diet that is plant based, with sufficient protein, is a key step toward supporting the depressed brain. Foods that are pro-inflammatory or do not provide the necessary nutrients will only contribute to depression. In fact, studies have shown that the typical Western diet with highly processed foods, high fats, and high carbohydrate is associated with higher levels of depression, while a growing number of studies have shown that plant-based diets, including the Mediterranean Diet, are associated with reduced levels of depression.

Among the popular diets, the Mediterranean Diet provides the right nutrients and fats for your brain. Its healthy forms of fat are particularly anti-inflammatory and help support the integrity of neurons because they are part of cellular membranes. In addition, eating foods that are low in simple carbohydrates versus the complex ones in most vegetables and some grains may prevent mood swings associated with rapid changes in the body's sugar levels. The main obstacle in trying to take up this diet while you are feeling down is that a depressed brain typically triggers your body to find comfort in part by craving sugars, starches, and processed foods that increase feel-good blood sugar levels. This is why when you get depressed, you turn to chocolate, candy, ice cream, and other high-carb foods. That is a big concern: the sugars will work for only a brief period of time and will deplete your system and cause you more trouble. Your brain has the right idea, but the wrong execution. In fact, patients with depression are more likely to become obese due to poor food choices, increased caloric intake, and decreased physical activity. Foods that are high in saturated fats and their various chemical constituents, like chips and pizza, are also common cravings of a depressed brain and can be big contributors to the inflammation that fuels the underlying depression.[2] Hence, the ideal foods are high-energy ones, such as green plants, which are anti-inflammatory due to their protein structures, and ones that have anti-inflammatory fats such as omega-3s found in fresh fish and omega-9s in olive oil.

Another diet-related aspect of depression has to do with the bacteria that live in your gut. The gut microbiome part of your brain-gut connection appears to have a great deal to do with your mood. When you have a healthy balance of bacteria in your gut, you reduce inflammation in your body, and that leads to improvements in the way your brain functions. A growing number of studies demonstrate that taking probiotics to improve the microbial balance in the gut may support a healthier mood.

Exercise is also essential for optimal brain function and improved mood. However, depression is often associated with lethargy and decreased motivation, which dampens the desire to be kinetic and thus will typically make you want to exercise even less. This frustrating cycle also contributes to the vicious cycle of inflammation because being sedentary leads to increased body fat, and that fat secretes excess inflammatory molecules which—you guessed it, worsen depression. Hence, the data showing a relationship between being obese and being depressed are growing. While it can be difficult, it is important for you to push through any lack of interest in exercising, even if it is just making yourself take a walk outside. In fact, two randomized clinical trials found exercise to be as good as antidepressant medications.[3] Other studies show that a combination of exercise and medication is superior to medication alone, including in patients with severe depression.[4] And if you can put together an integrative approach combining diet, exercise, and stress-reduction tools, along with medications when needed, there is potentially a much greater antidepressant effect.

MIND-BODY INTERVENTIONS

A variety of mind-body practices have been shown to be quite helpful in patients with depression. The mindfulness-based stress reduction program (MBSR) has often been shown to reduce depressive symptoms. We believe this may be due in large part to its facilitating nonjudgmental awareness, which then allows for a more objective appraisal of the negative cognitions and emotions associated with a depressed mood. It also requires engagement with others, which might help with breaking out of the social isolation that can be part of a depressed mood.

Because of the benefits of mindfulness, several psychotherapeutic approaches, such as cognitive behavioral therapy, have incorporated mindfulness into their programs as a way to more effectively alleviate symptoms of depression. And combining this type of mind-body approach, even with antidepressants, can be synergistic and potentially more effective than either approach alone.

A few studies have explored the specific effect of yoga practices in patients with depression, and overall, it appears that yoga and yoga meditation may be beneficial. Interestingly, one study with yoga instructors found that weekly yoga sessions resulted in increased alpha waves in the brain making them more relaxed and decreased cortisol in the body making them less stressed.[5] Thus, yoga can have some helpful effects important for achieving a balanced mood.

Acupuncture works by theoretically balancing the energy, or *qi* (also known as *chi*), in the body. This seems to make a lot of sense for treating depression in which brain energy is too low or imbalanced. Overall, a large number of studies have demonstrated that for the right person, acupuncture can be helpful for significantly reducing depressive symptoms with few, if any, side effects. One research conundrum, though, is that acupuncture typically has to be individualized, which makes it difficult to study and administer in a consistent manner. However, as with the other mind-body interventions, it can be a potential approach to consider.

SPIRITUALITY

As we have already discussed in detail, engaging in spiritual practices has big positive effects on your brain health. Research has also suggested that spiritual and religious practices may specifically have potent antidepressant benefits. For example, a number of studies have shown that those who view themselves as more religious or spiritual have lower levels of depression. And studies with a prospective approach have found that religious activity is associated with remission of depression in the future.[6] Dr. Lisa Miller from Columbia University has documented that religiousness in children and adolescents is highly protective against depression and suicide.[7] This pattern has also been found in adults, including the elderly. Though the degree of its impact is influenced by the person's social support, value of specific practices such as prayer, and inherent positive outlook associated with his or her particular religious beliefs.

With this in mind, some practitioners have successfully combined standard psychotherapy with religious elements to help patients turn to their religious beliefs as an added support for overcoming the depression. Thus, if you are a religious or spiritual person, seeking out those practices and paths during a time of depression can potentially be helpful. An interesting side note is that some people with depression have the opposite reaction: they expand their negative self-view outward to include religion and God.

SUPPLEMENTS AND DEPRESSION

Since symptoms of depression are so common, a large number of people who feel depressed look to supplements and botanicals to help alleviate their psychic pain. In fact, those with depression make up one of the largest groups of patients seeking complementary and alternative treatments. In part this is due to a large population with depression, but also because current medicines can be problematic and ineffective. And though finding something more "natural" has great appeal, it is important to remember that taking supplements needs to be thought of in the same way as taking medications. Their effectiveness can vary, and there can still be side effects or interactions with prescriptions. This is particularly true of herbs and botanicals that have medication-like effects versus taking extra of a naturally occurring substance like vitamin D that is already part of your body's biochemistry. Thus, it might be of value to consider basic vitamin repletion to ensure that vitamin deficiencies are not contributing to any depressive symptoms you may feel. We next provide an overview of some of the more common supplements.

St. John's Wort

St. John's wort (*Hypericum perforatum*) is a medicinal herb with antidepressant properties.[8] Several of its constituents, such as hypericum, hypericin, and hyperforin, also give antidepressant effects that appear to have a complex mechanism affecting the neurotransmitters serotonin, dopamine, and gamma-aminobutyric acid (GABA). A meta-analysis of thirty-seven double-blind randomized trials found that St. John's wort was equivalent to conventional antidepressant therapy for mild depression but less effective for severe depression.[9] But it needs to be considered as a medication, and it does interfere with the absorption or clearance of drugs including antiretrovirals, benzodiazepines, oral contraceptives, digoxin, phenobarbital, and theophylline.[10]

It is important to mention that while supplements with antidepressant effects such as St. John's wort and S-adenosyl-methionine can potentially be useful for the treatment of depressive symptoms, these supplements can also potentially induce manic symptoms in patients with bipolar disorder.[11] Caution is encouraged with complementary and alternative medicine (CAM) interventions that have been effective specifically for patients with depression, because they can potentially cause harmful effects in patients with bipolar disorder. Additionally, if combined with a number of serotonin-based antidepressants, a serious side effect, serotonin syndrome, can occur and can be life threatening. Again, it is always important to discuss and manage the use of St. John's wort and other supplements with your doctor.[12]

S-Adenosyl-Methionine

S-adenosyl-methionine (SAMe) is an amino acid important for the synthesis of neurotransmitters such as dopamine, norepinephrine, and serotonin. Studies have shown that it can be beneficial for those with depression, but probably not as a stand-alone therapy and certainly not for more severe conditions. Taking SAMe can also result in side effects such as insomnia or gastrointestinal problems. And some anti-Parkinsonian medications may have reduced effectiveness in patients who also take SAMe.

Omega-3 Fatty Acids

Omega-3 fatty acids have been shown to help as an adjunct therapy for managing depression. These fatty acids reduce inflammation and help neurons function more effectively. However, their effect is not strong enough by themselves to help with significant depressive symptoms. Also, having sufficient fatty acids in your diet might help protect from getting depression in the first place. Some clinical trials suggest that omega-3s could have an augmenting affect, thus making antidepressants more efficient.

Tryptophan and 5-Hydroxytryptophan

Some preclinical data suggest that tryptophan (TRP) and 5-hydroxytryptophan (5-HTP) may play a role in patients with depression, in part because both are amino acid precursors for serotonin. The overall results of a number of small studies of these compounds suggest that they help reduce symptoms in patients with major depressive disorder. The converse is also true: patients with depression are much more likely to relapse if they are on a tryptophan-depleted diet. So it is essential to have enough tryptophan in a diet, and taking it as a supplement might be a helpful way to do that for the right person.

CLINICAL TRIALS ON MOOD DISORDERS USING TARGETED NUTRIENTS

For serious mood disorders, such as major depression and bipolar disorder, psychiatric treatment is warranted. However, some clinical trials with patients with these conditions explored combining novel integrative approaches with standard medical care. For example, a small open-label trial demonstrated that oral magnesium supplementation might be useful in patients with rapid-cycling bipolar disorder.[13] A small case series also showed that intravenous magnesium sulfate could be used effectively along with standard medications in patients with bipolar disorder.[14] In addition, two small trials over six weeks showed that inositol worked as an adjunct to mood stabilizers.[15] Though no statistically significant changes were observed between the inositol and a placebo group, half of the participants in the inositol group did demonstrate a response. More data are required to determine whether inositol might be a useful adjunct therapy in treatments for bipolar patients.

A high prevalence of folic acid deficiency has been noted in some patients with depression and bipolar disorder, which suggests there may be a potential role for folic acid supplementation in these populations. One fifty-two-week trial of 102 patients with bipolar disorder who were already stabilized on lithium and also received either 200 milligrams of folic acid or a placebo showed significantly lower Beck Depression Inventory scores in the folic acid group.[16]

It has also been noted that populations in countries with high fish consumption have a lower prevalence of bipolar disorder, an observation that has led to several clinical trials that used omega-3 fatty acids in the treatment of bipolar patients.[17] Such studies have utilized fish oils and purified eicosapentaenoic acid (EPA) or docosahexaenoic acid (DHA). One trial that enrolled forty-four patients with bipolar disorder used a combination of EPA and DHA (9.6 grams per day) along with conventional drug therapies. Improvements in depressive symptoms were observed, but there was no significant effect on manic symptoms.[18] A small twenty-six-week open-label study showed that eight of ten participants treated with one month of EPA reported substantial improvements in their depressive symptoms.[19] A twelve-week study involving seventy-five patients with bipolar disorder, each of whom received 1 or 2 grams of EPA combined with standard psychiatric medication, demonstrated a small but significant improvement in depressive symptoms in the active groups but no observable changes in manic symptoms.[20] Other studies, including one of 121 patients, have demonstrated insignificant effects on symptoms of either depression or mania in bipolar patients.[21] One review article stated that the evidence weakly supports the use of omega-3 in combination with conventional medications in the depressive phase of bipolar disorder; however, omega-3 fatty acids do not appear to be effective in attenuating manic symptoms.[22]

Nutritional supplements with specific amino acids or nutrients have been used in the management of bipolar disorder. Two small, randomized studies have suggested that some branched-chain amino acids may improve acute mania by interfering with the synthesis of norepinephrine and dopamine. One study treated twenty-five patients with bipolar disorder with an oral blend of 60 grams per day of branched-chain amino acids such as leucine, isoleucine, and valine or a placebo. Participants in the amino acid group experienced significant reductions in the severity of their manic symptoms within six hours.[23] Furthermore, the symptom reductions were sustained with repeated administration of the branched-chain amino acids. Another study used N-acetyl cysteine (NAC), an amino acid with strong antioxidant properties, at a dose of 1 gram twice per day versus a placebo in seventy-five participants already stable in treatment for bipolar disorder. The findings indicated that NAC significantly reduced bipolar depression, yet no significant effect was observed on symptoms of mania.[24]

A separate review of eighteen randomized controlled trials reached similar conclusions about the use of various supplements for treating bipolar disorder.[25] In bipolar depression, NAC and a chelated mineral and vitamin formula were both shown to reduce depressive symptoms. Also, a chelated mineral formula of L-tryptophan, magnesium, folic acid, and branched-chain amino acid formulations all appeared to reduce manic symptoms in bipolar patients. The report indicated overall positive but still mixed evidence for omega-3 fatty acids in the treatment of depressive symptoms in bipolar disorder but found no supporting evidence for it in the management of manic symptoms.

It is important to mention that while supplements with antidepressant effects such as St. John's wort or SAMe can be useful for the treatment of depressive symptoms, these supplements can also potentially induce manic symptoms in patients with bipolar disorder.[26] Caution is encouraged with CAM interventions that have been effective specifically for patients with depression as they can potentially cause harmful effects in patients with bipolar disorder.

NEWER APPROACHES FOR DEPRESSION

One of the newest approaches for dealing with depression has been using some of the oldest drugs that fall under the category of psychedelics. For those alive in the 1960s, "magic mushrooms" and "acid" (LSD) were pretty available. For the last thirty years, because psychedelics were considered dangerous, they were illegal to use and certainly not considered in any kind of clinical setting.

But about ten years ago, several high-level researchers began to explore the impact they have on the brain and psyche. Their studies showed that psilocybin, the compound in magic mushrooms, had a significant effect on the serotonin system and produced intense "trips" comparable to spiritual experiences.[27] LSD has a similar impact on the serotonin system, which yields its potent hallucinogenic properties. A survey study we have performed over the past ten years directly compares descriptions of psychedelic experiences to more "natural" spiritual experiences and so far has found a great many similarities in their content and intensity. Researchers at Johns Hopkins have also found that the experiences under the influence of psilocybin are among the most powerful and transformative ones a person can have.[28] Since that time, these drugs have slowly been introduced into more clinical research, and the results have been quite amazing.

While more evidence is required, the initial results suggest that after one or two doses of a drug like psilocybin, those with depression have marked improvement in their symptoms. These improvements appear to be persistent, lasting for at least six months and maybe longer.[29] It is certainly compelling to think about using a drug only once or twice as a therapeutic approach for depression. This would eliminate a lot of the side effects of traditional antidepressants and likely come at a much-reduced cost. Of course, these compounds have their own potential side effects. People have certainly had "bad trips" on drugs like LSD, and there is the worry of addiction. However, the hope is that by administering these hallucinogens in a controlled therapeutic setting with a trained psychiatrist or therapist, they will be more effective and lead to positive outcomes.

Another drug, ketamine, has also been around for a long time, though as an anesthetic. Some early work with ketamine suggested that it may be able to reproduce near-death experiences in certain individuals. More recently, ketamine has been widely used to treat patients with migraines: findings have shown a substantial improvement in their pain symptoms. But it was also noted that migraine sufferers who received ketamine showed a reduction in their depressive symptoms as well. Ketamine is typically given as an inpatient intravenous infusion spread over four or five days for a period of about an hour or two each time. Others use a dosing regimen that spreads it out over a few weeks and in an outpatient setting. Ketamine does have its own side effects, including bad experiences resulting from overanxiousness. It remains to be seen whether ketamine and drugs like psilocybin will end up being part of the common treatments for depression. Since they also have problems with addiction and long-term consequences, it is too early to recommend them. Nevertheless, they are certainly something to keep an eye on.

In chapter 13, we considered several alternative approaches that have been shown to improve depressive symptoms. Neurofeedback can help to entrain the brain into a different pattern of activity with the goal of balancing that activity to reduce concerns like depression. But it typically takes fifteen to twenty sessions about once or twice a week to see meaningful results. Also, transcranial magnetic stimulation and direct current transcranial stimulation are ways to help modify brain function. Both have been shown to have beneficial effects in patients with depression by increasing activity in their key brain regions and more effectively balancing their brain activity.

Many patients with nonclinical depression can improve brain function through a number of other integrative and lifestyle modalities, several of which have been tested to document their benefits. For those with a clinically significant mood disorder, these approaches can still be useful adjuncts. And while medications appear to be effective for a number of patients with depressive disorders, at least one-third do not have a good response. In addition, antidepressants are drugs that have real side effects, so alternative strategies for mild depression—the kind that everyone experiences from time to time—are important to consider. Since inflammation is an important mechanism known to fuel depression, we encourage natural, integrative approaches to lowering systemic inflammation, such as optimal diet and nutrition, nutritional and botanical supplements, mind-body practices, and spiritual practices. Although more studies are needed across all of these domains, many of these methods are relatively safe and contribute to good brain health. Improving mood is part of weaving together a healthy brain, so we encourage you to work with your health care providers to maximize your available options.

Chapter 16
HEADACHES AND MIGRAINES

*All of us who have migraine suffer not only from the attacks
themselves but from this common conviction that we are perversely
refusing to cure ourselves by taking a couple of aspirin, that we are
making ourselves sick, that we "bring it on ourselves."*

—JOAN DIDION, 1968

Finding optimal ways to manage headaches and migraines is challenging; many hospitals have entire centers devoted to their treatment. Yet many people continue to have substantial symptoms that affect the way their brain works, daily living, and overall quality of life.

One of the first hurdles with the management of headaches is trying to figure out what is causing them. Part of this is based on the difficulty in arriving at a diagnosis. There are many different types of headaches: stress headaches, eyestrain headaches, tension headaches, cluster headaches, and an entire array of migraine headaches. Within the category of migraines, there can be typical migraines, episodic migraines, ocular migraines, vestibular migraines, and even migraines that affect the gastrointestinal tract instead of the brain. And even once an adequate diagnosis can be made, the physiology underlying any of them continues for the most part to elude medical science. For example, if you have migraines, we have an understanding that there is some type of alteration in your blood flow associated with your headaches. And though we have developed medical therapies that can specifically affect your blood flow in a positive way to help you feel fewer symptoms, we don't really know why the alterations in blood flow have this kind of an effect.

Another difficulty with headaches is associated with the bigger picture related to pain. When it comes to this, researchers have learned that pain has many components, and each of them may need to be addressed individually. To begin, there is the experience of the pain itself. Often patients are asked on a scale of 1 to 10, with 10 being the worst imaginable, to rate their pain. But not everyone's 7 is the same, and it is sometimes difficult to know their actual pain because it is subjective and some people are more stoic than others. Thus, beyond the biological pain itself are all of your emotional reactions to it. And finally, there is the impact of the limitations your pain can create for you.

We think about how to help patients with headache manage their pain in several ways. First, there is managing the headache in the acute phase, which typically requires some way of eliminating it quickly. This often takes medications, but we also consider a few integrative approaches as well. Integrative approaches typically become more useful in the chronic phase of headaches when we try to find ways to prevent them from occurring in the first place. And then there is the issue of helping patients with refractory headaches—those who do not seem to respond to any kind of standard treatment.

In patients with chronic headaches, our integrative approaches are often combined with conventional medical care. For example, patients suffering from tension headaches can sometimes respond to antidepressant medications. But they may also respond well to biofeedback, relaxation training, cognitive behavioral therapy for stress, or even physical therapy to help them deal with various muscular issues around their head and neck. And sometimes they respond well not to one but to a combination of several of these.

For cluster headaches, treatments can include calcium channel blockers for prevention, or ergotamine, greater occipital nerve blocks, steroids, lithium, sphenopalatine ganglion blocks, vagal nerve stimulation, and high amounts of oxygen.

One of the important considerations for us in the context of integrative medicine is when to sometimes help our patients wean off an overuse of medications.

For example, it is useful to evaluate if they are on inappropriate opioid medications or other prescriptions that might have long-term consequences. And when we advise them to go off those medications, we also help them during their withdrawal and in managing their headaches. Weaning off any medications should always be done in consultation with the primary doctor who prescribed the original medication as well as any additional health care providers who might help with the weaning process to avoid worsening symptoms, withdrawal symptoms, and any adverse interactions with other medications.

If you have migraines, you already know that you have many different triggers and that there can be many different ways to try to protect against having subsequent ones. But when it comes to trying to avoid those future migraines, often the first order of business is to figure out from your past what your triggers have been and make a plan from there. Some lifestyle-change remedies can include avoiding certain foods, being careful around certain types of lighting such as fluorescent bulbs, getting regular sleep, exercising regularly, and managing stress appropriately. While there are certainly medications that can also be used, changes to your lifestyle can be equally effective.

DIET AND NUTRITION

Migraine headaches in the acute setting typically include medications and are best prescribed by your doctor; however, you also have a number of additional possible therapeutic interventions. One interesting integrative approach for migraines in the acute phase that derives from basic nutrients is intravenously injecting magnesium.[1] This has been particularly helpful for migraine sufferers who also have a strange feeling, called an an aura, that precedes the onset of the actual headache. Patients presenting to hospitals typically get a combination of fluids, magnesium, and specific abortive medications. Magnesium also can come in oral formulations and is frequently used in these patients as a preventative against future migraines. Since it is typically too difficult to determine whether a patient truly has a magnesium deficiency that might predispose him or her to migraines, it is much easier to simply give the magnesium orally. The main issue with this is the side effect of gastrointestinal symptoms, particularly soft bowel movements or diarrhea. But this is a fairly easy fix since the oral dose can be titrated so that it does not cause adverse symptoms, and we hope proves to be beneficial.

Coenzyme Q10 (CoQ10), which helps increase energy production in the energy-producing part of the cell named the mitochondria, also appears to be potentially beneficial for treating migraines by possibly improving the energy production in the muscles and brain itself. A small randomized trial that gave 100 milligrams of CoQ10 three times per day was shown to be significantly more effective at preventing migraines than a placebo.[2] The vitamin riboflavin, also known as vitamin B2, is similarly involved in energy production, and has also been shown to be more effective than a placebo in patients with migraines when given as 400 milligrams per day.

Finally, there have been a number of attempts to modify diets as an approach to helping reduce migraine symptoms. Our Think Better Diet described in chapter 2 is similar to the Mediterranean Diet; however, ours is likely to be more beneficial for reducing migraines since diets high in plant-based foods with good oils and protein have been shown to be effective treatments for headaches.[3] Other dietary approaches have also been explored. For example, one study of approximately 150 patients suggested that the Ketogenic Diet may provide effective prophylaxis for chronic migraine sufferers. It is also essential that you be aware of various foods or food products that might trigger your migraines. Caffeine, MSG, aspartame, gluten, and histamine found in foods in general and other compounds found specifically in processed foods can all potentially make your migraines and other types of headaches worse.

An elimination diet can be particularly useful too when a number of food products seem to be triggers for your headaches.[4] Since spending three to four weeks on an elimination diet is relatively easy and free, it may be worthwhile to try and determine which foods are the culprits and then eliminate them. If there is no improvement through an elimination diet, then the cause of your headaches is something other than those food sources, which means you can then turn to other approaches, both conventional and integrative.

MIND-BODY PRACTICES

From an integrative medicine perspective, we would continue to use all options available to help you manage your headaches. This often starts with mind-body practices with the goal of reducing the stress and anxiety associated with headaches. That is because once you begin to feel a headache coming on, your stress and anxiety about the severity and ultimate outcome are enough to catapult your headache into a much more problematic issue. Practices like mindfulness and other meditation-based programs can be helpful in calming your reaction to your headache onset. Research has shown these programs can reduce the number and severity of headaches, even in patients with migraines.[5] Mindfulness can be also combined with cognitive therapy to help reduce stressors that might bring on migraine or tension-type headaches.

Physical exercise, which we have also discussed as always being essential to good brain health, has been found as well to be quite useful for reducing headache symptoms and their frequency. In particular, rigorous aerobic exercise approximately forty minutes per day, three to four times per week, seems to be especially good at reducing the frequency, intensity, and duration of migraines.[6] Exercising to relieve the stress causing tension headaches seems to be quite effective as well. Of course, some people's headaches can become worse with exercise, so be sure to assess your own strengths and weaknesses to determine whether exercising when you have a headache is right for you. Furthermore, while high-intensity training appears to be more effective, even more mild exercise, including mind-body practices such as yoga or tai chi, can be beneficial.

Massage can be beneficial too. In fact, several meta-analysis reviews have shown that massage can reduce migraine frequency by approximately 30 percent.[7] Chiropractic treatment, as well as osteopathic approaches to help better align the head and neck, have been shown to sometimes be useful. Various manual therapies have also frequently been used to help with menstrual headaches.

A number of studies, as well as a meta-analysis of more than fifteen hundred patients, have shown that biofeedback was more effective than a placebo for helping patients with tension-type headaches.[8] This means that modifying your body's response to stressors, including the pain from your headaches, appears to be helpful for reducing the number and intensity of headaches.

Several other randomized trials have shown that hypnosis can help reduce migraine frequency and symptoms.[9] Self-hypnosis training has been shown to decrease the severity of headaches as well as reduce the use of taking medication for them, while guided imagery training has been shown to help reduce the perception of the headache pain itself.

ADDITIONAL APPROACHES

An ancient approach to the management of headaches comes in the form of acupuncture. A large number of research studies have demonstrated that acupuncture can be quite beneficial for treating patients with headaches, including those with migraines.[10] If this sounds interesting to you, it is important that you see an experienced practitioner who can evaluate all aspects of your wellness and determine the appropriate acupuncture approach for you. Typically, if acupuncture is not helping within a couple of weeks, it is probably not going to be effective in the long run. Nevertheless, you might find great relief from it. We did some of the early research using single photon emission computed tomography (SPECT imaging) that demonstrated the impact acupuncture has on the brain's blood flow. We found that acupuncture alters activity in the pain pathways in a beneficial way so that the symptoms begin to resolve.[11]

Various brain stimulation therapies have also been effective in patients with headaches, including transcutaneous supraorbital nerve stimulation (tSNS), external vagus nerve stimulation (VNS), and occipital nerve transcutaneous electrical nerve stimulation (tONS). Each tries to stimulate nerves in certain ways in order to block pain transmission.

NATURAL PRODUCTS AND BOTANICALS

Medications to help with headaches range from the simple aspirin or ibuprofen to complex drugs like those we've discussed with wide-ranging effects on neurotransmitters, pain pathways, and perception of the pain itself. It is essential to talk with your doctor about these, as well as some of the other emerging treatments such as botox.

Botox injections around the forehead, temporal area, and occipital region have been shown to be particularly effective for those with chronic migraines; however, they are not as useful for episodic migraines.[12] Botox basically is a toxin that relaxes muscles, which appears to then help prevent migraine headaches.

You can also turn to a variety of natural products and supplements. Melatonin is a widely available supplement typically used for sleep; however, a few small studies have shown that 3 milligrams a day for migraines may be more effective than a placebo. It may even be as effective as the antidepressant amitriptyline.[13]

The botanical butterbur (*Petasites hybridus*) given as 75-milligram capsules, one to two times per day, has been shown to reduce the frequency of headaches.[14] A cautionary note is that a number of toxins that can lead to liver toxicity can be present in butterbur products. However, relatively pure products are considered to be safe.

Overall, migraines and other headache disorders are difficult to manage. But fortunately, the many available treatment options that include standard medications, dietary and nutritional modifications, mindfulness-based stress reduction, cognitive behavioral therapy, and other relaxation approaches have been shown to be quite useful. Thus, most people can find relief from these types of comprehensive integrative health programs in managing the many aspects of their headaches.

Chapter 17

CONCUSSIONS AND THE BRAIN

The brain is soft. Some of my colleagues compare it to
toothpaste, but that's not quite right. It doesn't spread like toothpaste.
It doesn't adhere to your fingers the way toothpaste does.
Tofu—the soft variety, if you know tofu—may be a more accurate
comparison. If you cut out a sizable cube of brain it retains its shape,
more or less, although not quite as well as tofu.

—Katrina Firlik, 2006

Concussion is a general term used to describe an injury to the head that affects the brain. Immediate symptoms may include headache, confusion, lack of coordination, memory loss, nausea, vomiting, dizziness, ringing in the ears, sleepiness, and excessive sleep. There may or may not be a loss of consciousness. Mild concussions often are self-resolving; however, we work with many patients who have long term post-concussive issues.

Concussions have been widely recognized as a substantial concern when it comes to brain health. Our brains may suffer multiple small traumas throughout our lives by falling on stairs, banging into an open cabinet, getting hit by a baseball, or even from the shaking of moderately violent amusement rides. No one really knows exactly how problematic all these minor injuries to the brain may be. The ones we do know about, though, are those specifically recognized as head injuries that lead to concussions. These are usually from more defined events such as a car accident, falling off a horse, or losing consciousness after colliding with someone in an ice hockey game.

The sports world has become highly engaged in the topic of concussion. The National Football League has particularly become involved in studying concussions, especially given the concern that the repetitive ones suffered by players can lead to the more devastating condition of chronic traumatic encephalopathy (CTE). The alarm about CTE is that it occurs on a cellular level, so it is often difficult to diagnose until clinicians can look at a person's brain after they die.

Concussions are a complex problem, with their effects ranging from the acute to chronic phase and resulting in a variety of potential health issues. So, how to best manage concussions is a big question. In the acute phase of a concussive head injury, a patient may experience an altered sense of consciousness or a loss of consciousness. In severe head injuries, such as in major car accidents or gunshot wounds, a large part of the brain may be physically altered to the extent that the patient can no longer maintain normal brain function and may even slip into a coma. These individuals often need acute care that can include surgery or support in an intensive care unit. While complete recovery is possible for them, they often need an extended period of time for substantial rehabilitation. Sometimes these patients have to relearn how to speak or understand language, or how to walk or use their hands, and often they have a substantial cognitive and emotional toll to deal with as well.

Others suffer what might be called mild concussions. In these circumstances, there is no obvious structural injury to their brain. In fact, most of their brain scans will look structurally normal, but that doesn't mean their brain is normal. What we have learned over the past thirty years by using high-tech imaging such as magnetic resonance imaging (MRI) and computerized tomography (CT) scanning to study the brains of patients who have had concussions is that there are tiny changes that markedly affect the neurons themselves and the connections between the neurons. Another concern with understanding the physiology of these head injuries is that no two are exactly alike. And because they often occur during sudden and unexpected accidents, it is virtually impossible to foresee how the injury will affect the brain and its functions.

Another variable is that every hit to the head can be slightly different in terms of the speed of impact; the angle; the direction the head moves, twists, and turns that the person might make to try to avoid the impact; and all the sloshing around the brain does inside the skull. On top of that, people go into a concussion with whatever brain they have up to that point. What we mean by this is that everyone has different genetics and different stages of brain development, some of which may make a person more prone to injury or more resistant to injury. It also means if you have had a prior concussion, how long ago it happened and how bad it was can influence your brain's recovery. Your diet and nutrition as well as any medications, alcohol, or recreational drugs you may have used can also have an impact on your resilience to the trauma. So when you go to your doctor with a concussion, it is going to be incredibly difficult to know exactly what the effects of that injury will be. A lot will also depend on your own strengths and weaknesses— more specifically, on the strengths and weaknesses of your cognitive and emotional functioning at the time of the concussion. If you already struggle with depression or with concentrating, you are vulnerable to those kinds of symptoms worsening. And if you have a strong cognitive reserve, it is likely your resilience will carry you through with a strongly functional brain.

The first piece of advice about concussions is an obvious one: try to avoid them. This means avoiding contact sports, being careful when driving, and wearing a helmet when cycling, skating, and doing other activities that could result in hitting your head. The other advice is also a preventive measure: try to keep your brain as healthy as possible every day throughout by following many of the guidelines we have already discussed" maintaining a healthy diet and weight, engaging in as many activities as possible, avoiding drugs and alcohol, getting the right amount of sleep, and reducing bad stress.

But if you have already had a concussion and continue to have symptoms now, what can you do about it?

In the short term after a concussion, most current recommendations say to rest your brain. That means to make sure you get enough downtime, refrain from using your brain vigorously such as at a busy workplace or school, and manage as best as possible any symptoms such as headaches. Though resting your brain can be beneficial for a few days, it is not recommended to rest it too long. Much like a muscle, if you rest your brain too much, it will start to become deconditioned. In fact, we even question the wisdom of resting the brain for extensive periods after concussions. For example, if you injure a muscle, you will rest it for a short period of time, but then it is important to slowly begin to exercise and stretch it again. Sometimes you may progress very slowly, but you want to keep working that muscle until it regains the strength it had before the injury. The same is true for your brain because it works in a similar way. You might need to take several days to truly rest your brain after a concussion, but then you should start engaging again very slowly, such as by reading, doing puzzles, talking to friends, or even watching some television, as long as none of those activities feel like they are over-whelming you or worsening your symptoms. If symptoms do begin to worsen, you need to stop that activity and most likely cut it back by a level or two before resuming. For severe brain injuries, patients need to work really hard at rehabilitation therapies that engage their brain on multiple levels to get the best results.

THE BRAIN AND CONCUSSIONS

At the Marcus Institute, we see a significant number of patients who continue to have symptoms even months or years after their concussion. These include headaches, light and sound sensitivities, cognitive impairments, emotional swings, dizziness and imbalance issues, and general brain fog. This has prompted us to initiate a large-scale study to explore what goes on in the brain of someone who has chronic symptoms from a concussion. This condition is also sometimes referred to as *post-concussive syndrome.* Most patients are frustrated when they come to see us because their scans and other diagnostic tests keep suggesting that everything is fine, even though they do not feel fine. From there we set out to do a much more robust job at exploring the effects of their concussion. Functional neuroimaging is one of the tools we have found to be particularly useful for this. There are a few ways of doing it, but one of the best is to use positron emission tomography (PET). A PET scan works by injecting a small amount of a radioactive tracer that helps us follow some part of the body's physiology. For the brain, one of the best tracers we have is fluorodeoxyglucose, a radioactive sugar taken up in the brain just like normal sugar is, from foods eaten, and allows us to observe whether there are areas of increased, normal, or decreased metabolic activity.

PET scans give us a functional picture of the brain and allow us to see which areas are working well and which are not. Interestingly, an overactive part of the brain or an underactive part can be equally detrimental to overall brain function. The analogy we use with our patients is to think of the brain as a car engine. Ideally, your engine works well by increasing its activity when you want to go faster and delivering more fuel into your engine. When you want to slow down, you take your foot off the pedal, less fuel gets into the engine, and you start to slow down. For example, when you are driving down the highway, the ideal is to have your engine in a nice balance that lets you speed up or slow down as you need to. The brain works in a similar way. When you are going through your everyday life, it is as if you're driving down the highway. If you suddenly need more activity from your brain to resolve a problem, more fuel, or in this case more sugar and oxygen, goes in, so that you are primed to find the answers you are looking for. And then when you are done with that particular activity, your fuel goes back to its baseline and your brain relaxes again.

But with concussions, one of two types of abnormalities can occur. Sometimes a brain area is just not working well, and this usually shows up as hypometabolism or as lower than normal activity on the PET scan.[1] This is like your car engine being unable to take in fuel or maybe is firing on only two cylinders instead of six. In the brain, this means that the neurons just aren't firing enough in a given part of the brain, such as the part involved in memory, which means memory will be impaired. The other abnormality involves overactivity in a particular area. This is somewhat like revving up your car engine while you have the emergency brake on. The engine wants to go, but something is stopping it from working the way it is supposed to. Similarly, in the brain, if an area is overactive or in a hypermetabolic state, then it is not able to work the way it is supposed to. For example, if the memory areas are already overactive, they can't increase their activity more when needed, and memory will be impaired. A PET scan is able to observe these kinds of changes and look at many different areas of the brain to see how they are working. In our ongoing study, we have found substantial abnormalities in the brains of patients who have post-concussive symptoms. We find areas of both increased and decreased metabolism that seem to correlate extremely well with the kinds of symptoms they are having. If a PET scan shows that their emotional centers are not operating normally, they typically are feeling distressing emotions such as depression or irritability.

Several other functional neural imaging approaches are available, one of which is single photon emission computed tomography (SPECT imaging) which has been made particularly well known by Dr. Daniel Amen through his extensive work with head injury patients, as well as patients with a variety of psychiatric concerns. This technique also involves injecting a small amount of a radioactive tracer in this case, one that follows blood flow in the brain. Just like our analogy with the car engine, blood flow is like fuel for your brain. SPECT is able to observe areas that are increased or decreased in response to patients who have a variety of brain conditions, most notably concussions.[2] For example, if a patient is not functioning well cognitively, then typically areas of this person's brain involved in memory and cognition are either overactive or underactive. The bigger question is how can we help fix these areas so that the patient can begin to function more effectively. We will get to that in a moment.

We also use another type of functional neuroimaging, functional magnetic resonance imaging (fMRI), to obtain various maps of functional processes in the brain. We use this technology as well in our study of patients with concussions. We have found that not only do they have abnormal function in the part of their brain that is injured, but also in the communication pathways between those injured parts and their other healthy brain structures. We have also found in the laboratory, under the microscope, that the injured brain part's nerve cells' connections are damaged. All of this corresponds to what we see clinically when different parts of the brain are not working well together. If different cognitive areas or emotional areas are not communicating well, we would expect our patients to have the kinds of symptoms that reflect the areas involved. We hope that our research will further the use of these functional imaging modalities and make them a more common approach to identifying areas of the brain affected by concussions.

RECOVERING FROM A CONCUSSION

Now we come to the most challenging and least understood aspects of the concussion: how to best manage it. As you might guess, we start by doing everything we can to minimize inflammation and oxidative stress in the system. Of course, a component of this is to optimize diet and nutrition. Eating a brain-healthy diet that reduces inflammation and is more plant-based with protein and plenty of healthy fats is always part of the plan. One of the arms of our research study has been to provide this type of nutritional counseling for our patients with post-concussive symptoms. We are encouraged by the results we have seen thus far. In fact, some of our patients have reported feeling that they had remarkable success just by improving their diet alone. Others have reported feeling mild improvements, and while this is anecdotal, it is terrific to be getting this kind of a positive signal from something that is relatively simple to incorporate into a treatment plan.

The next step is to find ways to improve brain function in the areas that are underactive and reduce the inflammation and overexcitation in the areas that are overactive. There are several ways to do this: some are nonmedicinal, some involve natural products, and some warrant medication.

Nonmedicinal approaches to improving post-concussive brain function typically come in the form of mind-body practices and neuromodulation techniques. In general, meditation practices can be extremely helpful for improving cognition and regulating emotions, including in those patients who have had a head injury.[3] While the data are not robust yet, since we know that meditation-based practices help reduce anxiety, stress, and depression and also help augment cognition, they are fundamental aspects of our brain health program. The main issue is that it has to be undertaken slowly. If you try a meditation practice and have too much trouble with it or if it is increasing your stress because it is too challenging, it is not right for you at that time. For example, it is possible that in the earlier stages, you might not be able to concentrate well, and so certain forms of concentrative meditation practices might be too difficult. But a few months down the road, if your brain is working better and you can concentrate better, that same meditation program might be quite rewarding.

Body movement is also important for recovering from a concussion. This can be in mild forms such as walking, tai chi, or yoga, or more moderate exercise, especially aerobics. Since exercise helps improve blood flow and function in the brain, it can be a valuable tool in helping to restore brain function after a concussion.[4] Again, be careful not overdo it, but if you are able, increase your exercise levels up as much as is reasonably possible.

Another nonmedicinal approach comes in the form of brain games and neuromodulation exercises.[5] Starting slowly with brain games as a way of exercising your brain after a concussion can be helpful in returning it to its original state of function. Again, much like a muscle, you want to do strengthening exercises for your brain as well. And as always, be careful not to overdo these either; if at any point you feel that you are overwhelming your brain's reserves or developing worsening symptoms, stop that practice and rest, and also think about alternative practices that might be better for you.

Neuromodulation and techniques such as neurofeedback can also be helpful in the right setting.[6] The goal of neurofeedback is to use your brain's electrical activities to help balance your brain's functions. As we have indicated, there are many areas of the brain that might be over- or underactive, which ultimately leads to an imbalance in neural functions. Although the data are rather limited, neurofeedback is often a part of our post-concussive program.

Transcranial magnetic stimulation (TMS) has also been used in patients with post-concussive symptoms. A benefit of it is that it can help enhance or reduce activity in certain parts of the brain. Combined with functional imaging, it may help rebalance the brain by augmenting areas that are underactive and by calming overactive areas . Several studies have demonstrated this to be an effective technique for helping patients recover from concussions, including improvements in their headache pain, depression, and cognition. One study even showed that of the patients treated with TMS, 60 percent of them returned to work, whereas only 10 percent in the control group did.[7]

Finally, some patients use natural products to help them recover from a concussion. Several on the market have unsupported claims, but one we feel is worth mentioning, even though the data are preliminary, is a strong antioxidant molecule, N-acetyl cysteine (NAC), which may help the brain by increasing levels of the body's own antioxidant molecule, glutathione. When an injury to the brain occurs, inflammation and oxidative damage occur at the cellular level, which can use up the body's glutathione stores. Thus, finding ways to restore glutathione may be beneficial for helping the healing process. NAC comes in both an intravenous and oral form. We have treated patients with both. The maximum impact seems to be in those who have intravenous infusions because that way, the NAC gets to high levels in the blood, which then may facilitate better glutathione levels. However, the oral form also seems to help a number of patients.

Our goal is to continue to improve diagnostic testing to determine whether a patient's condition has more to do with either the blood flow, metabolism, inflammation, or neurotransmitter imbalances and to continue to develop integrative and targeted therapies. In many ways, each patient ends up being his or her own experiment. Our road map includes a diet and nutritional program that minimizes inflammation and oxidative stress, increasing exercise and stress reduction, and then adding in a few of the specific therapies we've discussed. Brain injuries are challenging, but at the same time they present an incredible opportunity to use our unique integrative model to help a group of people who often are left with limited treatment options.

Chapter 18

COGNITIVE DISORDERS AND COGNITIVE ENHANCEMENT

Memory, of all the powers of the mind, is the most delicate and frail.

—BEN JOHNSON, 1641

Every year in the United States, there are more than 4.5 million adults with Alzheimer's disease, 3 million with Parkinson's disease, 1 million with other neurodegenerative disorders, and 800,000 with strokes. It goes without saying then that trying to find ways to help the brain deal with these devastating illnesses is at the forefront of much medical research. Until we have cures for these illnesses, and even after we find cures, it is imperative that you apply yourself to keeping your brain as healthy and resilient as possible for as long as possible. A recent article in the *Journal of the American Medical Association* stated that while "no medications have proven effective for [neurodegenerative disorders]; treatments and interventions should be aimed at reducing cardiovascular risk factors and prevention of stroke. Aerobic exercise, mental activity, and social engagement may help decrease risk of further cognitive decline."[1]

Thus, putting together a program to weave a tapestry of a healthy brain throughout your life is the best way you can protect your cognitive functions as you age. By focusing on the primary approaches we have already discussed—diet and nutrition, selected supplements, exercise, mind-body practices, social interactions, and spirituality—you can accomplish this. In addition, medications needed to keep other medical conditions such as thyroid disease, cholesterol, or high blood pressure under control are also important.

This last point deserves to be emphasized. The data on neurodegenerative diseases always implicate underlying risk factors such as high blood pressure, high cholesterol, thyroid issues, the metabolic syndrome, or diabetes mellitus particularly associated with obesity, physical inactivity, smoking, low vitamin D, low vitamin B_{12}, depression, taking too many medications, and untreated sleep apnea. All of these are risk factors for cognitive decline.[2] And they are all potentially treatable with many of the suggestions we give throughout this book. But sometimes medications are required. Please do not avoid medications because they are "unnatural" or "dangerous." Everything has a risk, including doing nothing. We always make sure our patients' overall health is optimized, and in our integrative model that sometimes requires medications. Of course, we also always seek to minimize the dosages and number of drugs by integrating lifestyle and wellness strategies.

Some medications can be quite helpful for your brain's functions. For instance, blood pressure medicines that help regulate the appropriate amount of blood to the brain are fundamental for brain health in patients with high blood pressure. Diuretics and centrally acting angiotensin enzyme inhibitors appear to reduce the lifetime risk of cognitive impairment and dementia, respectively.[3] And there is new evidence that statin cholesterol medicines appear to have direct neuroprotective effects.[4]

One of the main issues to consider is that most neurodegenerative processes and other injuries to the brain are associated with inflammation. The inflammatory process in the brain involves how oxidative stress occurs, how hormone imbalances happen, how different molecules are handled, how different proteins are processed, and how the many neurotransmitters and their receptors are balanced. Because of all of these potential factors, it is important to have a comprehensive plan that works on as many of them as possible.

DIET AND NUTRITION

You have likely figured out by now that diet and nutrition are essential for protecting your brain from cognitive decline and neurodegenerative disorders. We have shown throughout this book that the Think Better Diet, which is high in plant-based foods, adequate protein, rich in healthy fats from sources like fish and olive oil, and low in simple carbohydrates and saturated fats, is the most healthful one for your brain. A number of studies have shown how it helps reduce inflammation in your body and brain. So does the similar Mediterranean Diet and its modified version, which combines the Mediterranean Diet with the Dietary Approaches to Stop Hypertension (DASH) Diet, to create the Mediterranean-DASH Intervention for Neurodegenerative Delay Diet, more commonly know as the MIND Diet. Several studies have shown the MIND Diet to be quite helpful in reducing the risk of developing Alzheimer's and cognitive decline.[5]

Brain-healthy foods in the MIND Diet include vegetables, nuts, berries, beans, whole grains, fish, poultry, and olive oil. Brain-unhealthy foods include red and processed meats, butter and margarine, cheese, pastries and sweets, and fried and fast foods. General guidelines involve eating at least three servings of whole grains, a salad, one vegetable, and an optional single glass of wine per day. A serving of nuts each day can also be helpful, as can including beans as an excellent source of protein that is high in fiber and low in sugar.

In order to address concerns about cognitive decline or neurodegenerative disorders, it is vital that you maintain adequate levels of important nutrients. For example, your vitamin B12 levels positively correlate with your memory, concentration, and volume of the main memory area of your brain, the hippocampus. Hence, low vitamin B12 levels have been associated with cognitive decline. Other B vitamins, including folate, are essential nutrients for cellular processes, which means making sure you keep them at adequate levels through diet or additional supplementation,.

Vitamin D has a number of related functions, including offering neural anti-inflammatory and antioxidant effects, as well as neuroprotection by aiding in the clearance of abnormal proteins that have been found to contribute to neurodegenerative disorders.[6] And since most people are deficient in vitamin D, taking some amount as a supplement and monitoring your vitamin D levels to stay in the range of 40 to 50 international units (IU) per day may support your overall brain function and help protect you from neurodegenerative diseases. Most adult patients in our practice need to take at least 2000 IUs per day to maintain a healthy level. It is difficult to get enough vitamin D from food because the primary source for it is the sun. Yet we even find that patients who go outside regularly still often have low levels, probably because of sun blocks and other protective measures they wear to guard against skin cancer.

Vitamin E refers to eight lipid-soluble antioxidant compounds. In addition to functioning as antioxidants, there is evidence that vitamin E can also offer anti-inflammatory and neuroprotective benefits.[7] However, while low levels of this vitamin seem to be associated with reduced cognition, studies in which vitamin E supplementation was given have not been shown to particularly improve cognition or cognitive impairment.[8] One note of caution: vitamin E can cause blood thinning, so those on anticoagulants need to use vitamin E carefully.

Minerals such as magnesium and iron are important to regulate carefully as well. Too much or too little can be problematic for your brain and body. Magnesium is important for neuronal transmission, which means a magnesium supplement can be useful if you are deficient.

EXERCISE AND COGNITION

Being sedentary is a well-known risk factor for cognitive decline, and physical activity is well known for its strong neuroprotective effects. Exercise, especially aerobics, has been shown to improve blood flow to the brain and increase energy metabolism. Furthermore, exercise has been correlated with larger brain volumes, particularly in the hippocampus.[9] Physical activity is also associated with measurable improvements in memory, executive functioning, processing speed, and visuospatial skills. Stretching and resistance training are also beneficial, but probably not as much as aerobic exercise, at least with regard to your brain. What is most important is to create an exercise regimen that works for you. The many options range from the basic like walking to reclining bicycles to the sophisticated aquatherapy. Exercise is also important for helping your body function better, including by improving your balance and coordination to help you avoid falls, which can lead to concussions.

SLEEP AND COGNITION

It is always important for your brain to get the right amount of sleep. We mentioned in chapter 6 that there are a number of potential reasons for sleeplessness and ways to try to fix them. But we do want to emphasize that better sleep is associated with better cognition. For example, an eight-year study of patients with sleep apnea found that treatment with continuous positive airway pressure therapy slowed their decline in memory scores as they aged.[10] Both light therapy and melatonin have also been shown to promote a healthy sleep schedule. Furthermore, thirty minutes of ten thousand lux from a light box treatment (using the same light box deployed for adults with seasonal affective disorder) in the morning has been shown to reduce aggression in Alzheimer's disease patients.[11]

One of our own recent studies showed that poor sleep led to a greater accumulation of amyloid protein in the brain, the protein involved in Alzheimer's disease. Additionally, not sleeping well has been shown to contribute to poor cognition, mostly by causing a buildup of the amyloid. These results suggest that getting better sleep is important whether you are trying to avoid Alzheimer's or, sadly, have it.

MIND-BODY PRACTICES AND CHALLENGING YOUR BRAIN

We previously described how meditation and other mind-body practices have potential benefits for your brain health, including improving symptoms of depression and anxiety, as well as attention and cognition. We also discussed that a common mechanism for both depression and cognitive decline is inflammation, which our entire integrative approach is geared toward minimizing. There is some clinical overlap here too since it is well known that depression is associated with poor cognition. In fact, it can be difficult to distinguish some elderly patients with depression from those with diseases like Alzheimer's. The appearance of both can be similar, because these patients generally talk less, engage less often in activities, and seem to think less clearly. Practices that have dual positive effects on depression and cognition can be useful, and many mind-body practices do just that.

Meditation, mindfulness, Kirtan Kriya, yoga, tai chi, and many other like-minded approaches can be useful to cognitive functions. But the main issue is whether the individual can do the practice. If the cognitive impairment is so severe that it prevents being able to meditate, then it will not be helpful, and instead a program like yoga or tai chi might be better since the person can do the movements and still derive some benefit. Our studies, as well as those of a number of other investigators, have consistently shown that these practices change the way the brain functions and even the way it is structured. Since neurodegenerative diseases are associated with a loss of brain tissue, having more tissue to start with can be helpful. Meditation practices, done over long periods of time, have shown they can offer that. In fact, long-term meditators have larger brains, particularly in their frontal lobes.[12]

Adults doing a regular yoga practice have been found to have improved verbal abilities and increased function in brain regions related to verbal memory, language processing, and visuospatial memory.[13] A fair amount of data shows that yoga also improves psychological health by reducing depression and anxiety and enhancing well-being. As with exercise, yoga can improve balance and coordination, which becomes a plus for protecting the brain from accidents. Clearly, some form of mind-body practice can be helpful to protect the brain and cognitive powers.

The more you use your brain, the better are your chances of warding off cognitive decline. And one of the best ways to do that is through social engagement. Talking to others, arguing, loving, and all the ways in which we engage with other people have been shown to protect the brain from both normal aging and neurodegenerative disease.[14] Make sure you get out of the house, meet with your friends and family, attend spiritual or religious gatherings, go to cultural events, visit the zoo, have a poker night, go bowling, play a sport with others, attend a musical concert, or visit museums and art galleries. The goal is to place your brain in a socially and, ideally, intellectually stimulating environment. The more you do this, the more your brain will continue to absorb, adapt, and strengthen.

Spiritual and religious activities by themselves have been shown to be beneficial for your brain's overall health and function. More specifically, those who engage in regular religious and spiritual activities have a lower rate of neurodegenerative diseases.[15] Whether it is the social engagement, the meditation or prayer practices, or the positive outlook derived from a relationship with a higher power, if you have a strong spiritual side, it is helpful to actively engage with it. But one thing to look out for is something called "religious struggle." It can occur at any point in life, though frequently it arises in elderly individuals who have trouble getting to their house of worship or engaging in their tradition in the same way they had previously been able to. In these cases, they can sometimes become anxious because they are unable to nurture their beliefs properly, though consulting with someone from pastoral care or the clergy can still be helpful to comfort and support them.

We have already discussed different brain games for weaving together an overall healthy brain. As you confront various cognitive challenges, engaging in these activities can help stimulate and enhance your brain function. You can think of it this way: if a professional athlete were to stop training for a month, his or her skills and endurance would decline, and fairly quickly. With that in mind, strive to train your brain to engage in challenging tasks every day and in a variety of activities, including putting puzzles together, writing music, attending a play, listening to an interesting podcast, or reading a book. The more you do all of these activities, the more likely you will be to improve your brain's function and your quality of life. One important note to point out here is that passive mental activity, such as watching television, is not particularly beneficial for your brain. It can be helpful if it is a truly engaging, educational program, but otherwise, most health care providers recommend limiting watching television to no more than two hours per day

Cognitive training programs and apps have become widespread and popular. Doing any of these brain games typically improves your skills in that particular game rather than in a generalized cognitive way. However, doing a bunch of different ones may help improve different domains of your cognitive function and lead to more global improvements for you. If you are specifically interested in computerized training to enhance your cognition, the best thing to do is to consult with a neuropsychologist or occupational therapist who can help you choose the programs and tasks that will be best for you based on your strengths, limitations, and needs.

NUTRITIONAL SUPPLEMENTS FOR COGNITIVE DECLINE

There are many over-the-counter supplements that claim to benefit cognition and stave off dementia. Unfortunately, none of them have not been well tested or validated by the medical community or the Food and Drug Administration, though a recent meta-analysis found that several common supplements such as omega-3 fish oil, B vitamins, and vitamin E did not improve cognition in nondemented adults. That said, small studies have shown some of these over-the-counter supplements were beneficial and could be useful provided that they do not interfere with other medications or disease processes.

Although omega-3 fatty acids have not been shown to specifically improve cognition, they are well known to help reduce inflammation and to be essential elements of cell membranes. This suggests they might be better when used as part of a larger brain health program. For example, one study showed that omega-3 fatty acids taken in combination with aerobic exercise resulted in higher gray matter brain volumes in patients with mild cognitive impairment. Furthermore, patients who had high levels of omega-3 fatty acids in their diet tended to be at lower risk for cognitive impairment, so, it is important to make sure you get sufficient omega-3 fatty acids in your diet or through appropriate supplementation.

Phosphatidyl serine is a phospholipid that also makes up elements of cell membranes. It is commercially available as Vayacog, and in one small study patients who received it over a fifteen-week period showed improvement in memory and learning.[16]

We have performed several studies looking at N-acetylcysteine (NAC) and its function as a strong antioxidant in the brain. Our data have shown that it improves cognition in several patient populations. In particular, we have studied the impact of NAC in patients with multiple sclerosis, a disorder that destroys the connections between neurons. Using PET scans, we found that NAC particularly helps improve neuronal function and metabolism in the cognitive parts of the brain such as the temporal lobe even in patients with substantial brain injury from their illness.[17] You can see some of these results in the brain imaging figures titled Natural Supplement for Multiple Sclerosis Treatment in the color photography section. And one small study of Alzheimer's disease patients given NAC over a six-month period showed improvements in their cognitive performance.

Resveratrol, an antioxidant found in certain fruits and berries, appears to slow a variety of brain-related processes that can lead to neurodegeneration. It may reduce inflammation, mitochondrial dysfunction, and the formation of detrimental proteins such as amyloid. By reducing these processes, it is believed that it might protect against cognitive decline. Resveratrol has also been found to increase hippocampal function in healthy older adults.[18] It is important to note that it is generally well tolerated, but some people can have side effects such as fatigue, increased diastolic blood pressure, gastrointestinal symptoms, diarrhea, or weight loss.

Other compounds that function as antioxidants include polyphenols, which are found in a number of food sources such as pomegranates. One study found that people with mild memory loss who drank eight ounces of pure pomegranate juice daily for twenty-eight days had an increase in their memory, as well as higher activity in their thalamus and frontal lobes, two areas heavily involved in concentration and memory.[19] Other studies have shown that mice given pure pomegranate juice from ages six to twelve and a half months have cognitively outperformed those given sugar water.

NEUROMODULATORY APPROACHES

The neuromodulation techniques of transcranial magnetic stimulation (TMS) and direct current transcranial stimulation (tDCS) are now being looked at more actively as potential therapies for patients with cognitive impairments. The data for both technologies is still preliminary. In one study, patients with mild-stage Alzheimer's disease had significant improvements in memory and language scores after undergoing a TMS protocol that over a six-week period stimulated the frontal lobe and higher cognitive areas of the brain. Repetitive transcranial magnetic stimulation (rTMS), which is experimental and not FDA approved, when used in conjunction with cognitive training, was found to improve cognitive performance in a study of Alzheimer's patients.[20] Also, studies using tDCS in patients with Alzheimer's found improvements in their cognitive function over those who did not receive the stimulation.[21] More studies are needed to reveal to what degree these devices are appropriate for the clinical management of cognitive decline in patients or for those at risk of developing it.

NEUROGROW BRAINFITNESS PROGRAM

The NeuroGrow BrainFitness program is another integrative treatment combining cognitive skills training, counseling, meditation training, treatment for medical conditions including depression and sleep apnea, weekly neurofeedback, weekly cognitive stimulation, coaching and counseling for stress reduction, diet coaching, and exercise. Studies of this intervention over a twelve-week period found participants had improved cognitive function and brain growth in the hippocampus.[22]

INTEGRATING APPROACHES

You are your own brain weaver, and our goal is nothing short of empowering you with as many tools as possible to help you be the best one you can be. While there are environmental and genetic factors, there also are many things you can do to establish your resilience and dampen pathological processes. We emphasize a program that integrates multiple components such as diet and nutrition, mind-body practices, spirituality, and selected supplements, as well as medications when needed. While the medical world is slowly catching up to this idea, you can be on the cutting edge by taking a proactive stance. A growing body of literature supports this path. One in particular is the FINGER study, a randomized, controlled trial of several thousand at-risk elderly adults to study an intervention consisting of regular group meetings with a nutritionist, personally tailored physical exercise programs, and group and individualized cognitive training sessions.[23] After a two-year period, participants in the active arm experienced significant improvements in their executive functioning and processing speed, as well as better dietary habits and increased physical activity as compared to the placebo group. They also lost more weight.

All of these studies underscore the importance of what we've discussed to help you keep your brain healthy and functional for as long as you can. We encourage you to start anywhere you like on this journey—with diet, stress reduction, spirituality, or something else—and to keep layering on new health-promoting behaviors and lessons you learn along the way. The effort will make a difference, and your brain and body will thank you.

Epilogue
YOU ARE A BRAIN WEAVER

Our overarching goal for this book is to provide *you* the reader, *you* the weaver of your own brain, with the latest information about how your brain works and, more important, empower you with the right set of tools to achieve and maintain optimal brain health. The model we've developed at the Marcus Institute of Integrative Health at Thomas Jefferson University combines the four dimensions of life—the biological, psychological, social, and spiritual—and in a way that is guided by advanced scientific studies, many of which we have performed ourselves.

A key to your success is learning how to maximize your natural strengths while incorporating our proven strategies to face your challenges and thereby reduce deficits. This is a whole-life approach to the health of your brain and body arrived at by drawing on the scientific literature and our vast experience with numerous illness and wellness populations.

Everything you do and everything you experience affects the fabric of your brain. What you eat, what you think, how well you sleep, how you feel emotionally, your level of physical activity, and how well the rest of the systems in your body function all affect your brain's biology. You are a complex network of systems within systems, which underscores the importance of our bio-psycho-social-spiritual approach.

Biologically, it is of fundamental importance to protect your brain as best as possible by avoiding toxins, being cautious about physical injuries, and doing as many brain-stimulating activities as you can. It also is important to fuel your brain with the right nutrients and to minimize inflammation from junk foods, processed foods, and those with excess sugar.

Psychologically, it is critical during these stressful times we live in that a central objective be incorporating stress reduction into your daily life. We reviewed several proven strategies to help with this, including breathing techniques, focusing on positive emotions such as gratitude and compassion, and using meditation, the Neuro Emotional Technique, and other mind-body therapies. The pre- and post-brain scans and other metrics we have provided show just how transformative these approaches can be for you.

Socially, we reviewed how your brain is hardwired to connect with others. It is especially important during times of necessary social distancing that you find creative ways to engage with others. Your brain health, and overall health, suffers when you have too much isolation, loneliness, and decreased connection with the outside world. So find ways to learn from people, interact with them, and talk with them as much as possible. Having a strong social support network is important.

Spiritually, all of our research has shown that regularly engaging in activities that give us meaning has an incredible impact on the brain. You may find deep meaning in religious traditions, or in meditation practices, nature, or something else that feels sacred. You can also find spirituality by engaging the creative part of your brain in music, art, and other inspirations. Ultimately, finding meaning and purpose in your life, and living your life to the fullest, are perhaps the most important pillars for your healthy brain.

With this information, we humbly hope that you integrate at least a few of these tools into your daily life to go forward with your best brain possible. Nothing would make us happier. We wish you well on your journey.

ACKNOWLEDGMENTS

W e are thankful for the incredible partnership with the Marcus Foundation; the forward-thinking leadership of Thomas Jefferson University; and our mentors, colleagues, and patients who taught us along the way. We also have tremendous gratitude for our additional research partners, such as the Adolph Coors Foundation and the ONE Research Foundation.

NOTES

Chapter 2

1. Zhang, Lin, Dongxia Hou, Xi Chen, Donghai Li, Lingyun Zhu, Yujing Zhang, and Jing Li et al. 2011. "Exogenous Plant Mir168a Specifically Targets Mammalian LDLRAP1: Evidence of Cross-Kingdom Regulation by Microrna." *Cell Research* 22 (1): 107–126. doi:10.1038/cr.2011.158.

2. Dash, Sarah, Gerard Clarke, Michael Berk, and Felice N. Jacka. 2015. "The Gut Microbiome and Diet in Psychiatry." *Current Opinion in Psychiatry* 28 (1): 1–6. doi:10.1097/yco.0000000000000117; Francis, Heather, and Richard Stevenson. 2013. "The Longer-Term Impacts of Western Diet on Human Cognition and the Brain." *Appetite* 63: 119–128. doi:10.1016/j.appet.2012.12.018.

3. McGrattan, Andrea M., Bernadette McGuinness, Michelle C. McKinley, Frank Kee, Peter Passmore, Jayne V. Woodside, and Claire T. McEvoy. 2019. "Diet and Inflammation in Cognitive Ageing and Alzheimer's Disease." *Current Nutrition Reports* 8 (2): 53–65. doi:10.1007/s13668-019-0271-4; Solfrizzi, Vincenzo, Francesco Panza, Vincenza Frisardi, Davide Seripa, Giancarlo Logroscino, Bruno P. Imbimbo, and Alberto Pilotto. 2011. "Diet and Alzheimer's Disease Risk Factors or Prevention: the Current Evidence." *Expert Review of Neurotherapeutics* 11 (5): 677–708. doi:10.1586/ern.11.56.

4. Barnard, Neal D., Ashley I. Bush, Antonia Ceccarelli, James Cooper, Celeste A. de Jager, Kirk I. Erickson, and Gary Fraser et al. 2014. "Dietary and Lifestyle Guidelines for the Prevention of Alzheimer's Disease." *Neurobiology of Aging* 35: S74–S78. doi:10.1016/j.neurobiolaging.2014.03.033.

5. Lange, Klaus W. 2020. "Omega-3 Fatty Acids and Mental Health." *Global Health Journal* 4 (1): 18–30. doi:10.1016/j.glohj.2020.01.004.

6. Fritsche, Kevin L. 2015. "The Science of Fatty Acids and Inflammation." *Advances in Nutrition* 6 (3): 293S–301S. doi:10.3945/an.114.006940.

7. Pallazola, Vincent A., Dorothy M. Davis, Seamus P. Whelton, Rhanderson Cardoso, Jacqueline M. Latina, Erin D. Michos, and Sudipa Sarkar et al. 2019. "A Clinician's Guide to Healthy Eating for Cardiovascular Disease Prevention." *Mayo Clinic Proceedings: Innovations, Quality & Outcomes* 3 (3): 251–267. doi:10.1016/j.mayocpiqo.2019.05.001.

8. Shahidi, Fereidoon, and Priyatharini Ambigaipalan. 2018. "Omega-3 Polyunsaturated Fatty Acids and Their Health Benefits." *Annual Review of Food Science and Technology* 9 (1): 345–381. doi:10.1146/annurev-food-111317-095850.

9. Torres, Nimbe, Martha Guevara-Cruz, Laura A. Velázquez-Villegas, and Armando R. Tovar. 2015. "Nutrition and Atherosclerosis." *Archives of Medical Research* 46 (5): 408–426. doi:10.1016/j.arcmed.2015.05.010.

10. Calder, Philip C., Nabil Bosco, Raphaëlle Bourdet-Sicard, Lucile Capuron, Nathalie Delzenne, Joel Doré, and Claudio Franceschi et al. 2017. "Health Relevance of the Modification of Low Grade Inflammation in Ageing (Inflammageing) and the Role of Nutrition." *Ageing Research Reviews* 40: 95–119. doi:10.1016/j.arr.2017.09.001.

11. Murata, Masaharu, and Jeong-Hun Kang. 2018. "Bisphenol A (BPA) and Cell Signaling Pathways." *Biotechnology Advances* 36 (1): 311–327. doi:10.1016/j.biotechadv.2017.12.002.

12. Wang, Xia, Xinying Lin, Ying Y. Ouyang, Jun Liu, Gang Zhao, An Pan, and Frank B. Hu. 2015. "Red and Processed Meat Consumption and Mortality: Dose–Response Meta-Analysis of Prospective Cohort Studies." *Public Health Nutrition* 19 (5): 893–905. doi:10.1017/s1368980015002062.

13. Vigar, Vanessa, Stephen Myers, Christopher Oliver, Jacinta Arellano, Shelley Robinson, and Carlo Leifert. 2019. "A Systematic Review of Organic Versus Conventional Food Consumption: Is There a Measurable Benefit on Human Health?" *Nutrients* 12 (1): 7. doi:10.3390/nu12010007.

14. Shapira, Niva. 2019. "The Metabolic Concept of Meal Sequence vs. Satiety: Glycemic and Oxidative Responses with Reference to Inflammation Risk, Protective Principles and Mediterranean Diet." *Nutrients* 11 (10): 2373. doi:10.3390/nu11102373.

Chapter 5

1. Li, Nannan, Qi Wang, Yan Wang, Anji Sun, Yiwei Lin, Ye Jin, and Xiaobai Li. 2019. "Fecal Microbiota Transplantation from Chronic Unpredictable Mild Stress Mice Donors Affects Anxiety-Like and Depression-Like Behavior in Recipient Mice via the Gut Microbiota-Inflammation-Brain Axis." *Stress* 22 (5): 592–602. doi:10.1080/10253890.2019.1617267.

2. Butel, M.-J. 2014. "Probiotics, Gut Microbiota and Health." *Médecine et Maladies Infectieuses* 44 (1): 1–8. doi:10.1016/j.medmal.2013.10.002.

3. Akkasheh, Ghodarz, Zahra Kashani-Poor, Maryam Tajabadi-Ebrahimi, Parvaneh Jafari, Hossein Akbari, Mohsen Taghizadeh, et al. 2016. "Clinical and Metabolic Response to Probiotic Administration in Patients with Major Depressive Disorder: A Randomized, Double-Blind, Placebo-Controlled Trial." *Nutrition* 32 (3): 315–320. doi:10.1016/j.nut.2015.09.003.

4. Zeng, M. Y., N. Inohara, and G. Nuñez. 2016. "Mechanisms of Inflammation-Driven Bacterial Dysbiosis in the Gut." *Mucosal Immunology* 10 (1): 18–26. doi:10.1038/mi.2016.75.

5. NIH Human Microbiome Project. 2009. *Microbe Magazine* 4 (9): 393–393. doi:10.1128/microbe.4.393.1.

6. Hildebrandt, Marie A., Christian Hoffmann, Scott A. Sherrill–Mix, Sue A. Keilbaugh, Micah Hamady, Ying–Yu Chen, et al. 2009. "High-Fat Diet Determines the Composition of the Murine Gut Microbiome Independently of Obesity." *Gastroenterology* 137 (5): 1716–1724. e2. doi:10.1053/j.gastro.2009.08.042.

7. Milner, J. Justin, and Melinda A. Beck. 2012. "The Impact of Obesity on the Immune Response to Infection." *Proceedings of the Nutrition Society* 71 (2): 298–306. doi:10.1017/s0029665112000158.

8. Cheung, Stephanie G., Ariel R. Goldenthal, Anne-Catrin Uhlemann, J. John Mann, Jeffrey M. Miller, and M. Elizabeth Sublette. 2019. "Systematic Review of Gut Microbiota and Major Depression." *Frontiers in Psychiatry* 10. doi:10.3389/fpsyt.2019.00034.

9. Li, Nannan, Qi Wang, Yan Wang, Anji Sun, Yiwei Lin, Ye Jin, and Xiaobai Li. 2019. "Fecal Microbiota Transplantation from Chronic Unpredictable Mild Stress Mice Donors Affects

Anxiety-Like and Depression-Like Behavior in Recipient Mice Via the Gut Microbiota-Inflammation-Brain Axis." *Stress* 22 (5): 592–602. doi:10.1080/10253890.2019.1617267.

10. Burokas, Aurelijus, Silvia Arboleya, Rachel D. Moloney, Veronica L. Peterson, Kiera Murphy, Gerard Clarke, et al. 2017. "Targeting the Microbiota-Gut-Brain Axis: Prebiotics Have Anxiolytic and Antidepressant-Like Effects and Reverse the Impact of Chronic Stress in Mice." *Biological Psychiatry* 82 (7): 472–487. doi:10.1016/j.biopsych.2016.12.031.

11. Braniste, V., M. Al-Asmakh, C. Kowal, F. Anuar, A. Abbaspour, M. Toth, and A. Korecka et al. 2014. "The Gut Microbiota Influences Blood-Brain Barrier Permeability in Mice." *Science Translational Medicine* 6 (263): 263ra158-263ra158. doi:10.1126/scitranslmed.3009759.

Chapter 4

1. Centers for Disease Control and Prevention. Fourth Report on Human Exposure to Environmental Chemicals, 2009. Atlanta, GA: U.S. Department of Health and Human Services, Centers for Disease Control and Prevention. 2021. *Cdc.Gov*. https://www.cdc.gov/exposurereport/pdf/fourthreport.pdf.

2. Dauer, William, and Serge Przedborski. 2003. "Parkinson's Disease." *Neuron* 39 (6): 889–909. doi:10.1016/s0896-6273(03)00568-3.

3. Kales, Stefanos N., and Rose H. Goldman. 2002. "Mercury Exposure: Current Concepts, Controversies, and a Clinic's Experience." *Journal of Occupational and Environmental Medicine* 44 (2): 143–154. doi:10.1097/00043764-200202000-00009.

4. Spencer, A. J. 2000. «Dental Amalgam and Mercury in Dentistry." *Australian Dental Journal* 45 (4): 224–234. doi:10.1111/j.1834-7819.2000.tb00256.x.

5. Galvano, Fabio, Andrea Piva, Alberto Ritieni, and Giacomo Galvano. 2001. "Dietary Strategies to Counteract the Effects of Mycotoxins: A Review." *Journal of Food Protection* 64 (1): 120–131. doi:10.4315/0362-028x-64.1.120.

6. Hussain, Joy, and Marc Cohen. 2018. "Clinical Effects of Regular Dry Sauna Bathing: A Systematic Review." *Evidence-Based Complementary and Alternative Medicine* 2018: 1–30. doi:10.1155/2018/1857413.

7. Sultan, Sulaiman, Shishir Murarka, Ahad Jahangir, Farouk Mookadam, A. Jamil Tajik, and Arshad Jahangir. 2017. "Chelation Therapy in Cardiovascular Disease: An Update." *Expert Review of Clinical Pharmacology* 10 (8): 843–854. doi:10.1080/17512433.2017.1339601.

8. Cuajungco, Math P., Kyle Y. Faget, Xudong Huang, Rudolph E. Tanzi, and Ashley I. Bush. 2006. "Metal Chelation as a Potential Therapy for Alzheimer's Disease." *Annals of the New York Academy of Sciences* 920 (1): 292–304. doi:10.1111/j.1749-6632.2000.tb06938.x.

9. Sears, Margaret E. 2013. "Chelation: Harnessing and Enhancing Heavy Metal Detoxification—A Review." *Scientific World Journal* 2013: 1–13. doi:10.1155/2013/219840.

10. Mastinu, Andrea, Amit Kumar, Giuseppina Maccarinelli, Sara Anne Bonini, Marika Premoli, Francesca Aria, et al. 2019. "Zeolite Clinoptilolite: Therapeutic Virtues of an Ancient Mineral." *Molecules* 24 (8): 1517. doi:10.3390/molecules24081517.

11. Rea, William J. 2018. "A Large Case-Series of Successful Treatment of Patients Exposed to Mold and Mycotoxin." *Clinical Therapeutics* 40 (6): 889–893. doi:10.1016/j.clinthera.2018.05.003.

Chapter 5

1. Newberg, Andrew B., Nancy Wintering, Dharma S. Khalsa, Hannah Roggenkamp, and Mark R. Waldman. 2010. "Meditation Effects on Cognitive Function and Cerebral Blood Flow in Subjects with Memory Loss: A Preliminary Study." *Journal of Alzheimer's Disease* 20 (2): 517–526. doi:10.3233/jad-2010-1391.

2. Greydanus, Donald E., Helen D. Pratt, and Dilip R. Patel. 2007. "Attention Deficit Hyperactivity Disorder across the Lifespan: The Child, Adolescent, and Adult." *Disease-a-Month* 53 (2): 70–131. doi:10.1016/j.disamonth.2007.01.001.

3. Froeliger, Brett, Eric L. Garland, and F. Joseph McClernon. 2012. "Yoga Meditation Practitioners Exhibit Greater Gray Matter Volume and Fewer Reported Cognitive Failures: Results of a Preliminary Voxel-Based Morphometric Analysis." *Evidence-Based Complementary and Alternative Medicine* 2012: 1–8. doi:10.1155/2012/821307.

4. Au, Jacky, Ellen Sheehan, Nancy Tsai, Greg J. Duncan, Martin Buschkuehl, and Susanne M. Jaeggi. 2014. "Improving Fluid Intelligence with Training on Working Memory: A Meta-Analysis." *Psychonomic Bulletin & Review* 22 (2): 366–377. doi:10.3758/s13423-014-0699-x; Nahum, Mor, Hyunkyu Lee, and Michael M. Merzenich. 2013. "Principles of Neuroplasticity-Based Rehabilitation." *Changing Brains: Applying Brain Plasticity to Advance and Recover Human Ability*, 141–171. doi:10.1016/b978-0-444-63327-9.00009-6.

5. Wentink, M. M., M. A. M. Berger, A. J. de Kloet, J. Meesters, G. P. H. Band, R. Wolterbeek, P. H. Goossens, and T. P. M. Vliet Vlieland. 2016. "The Effects of an 8-Week Computer-Based Brain Training Programme on Cognitive Functioning, QoL and Self-Efficacy after Stroke." *Neuropsychological Rehabilitation* 26 (5–6): 847–865. doi:10.1080/09602011.2016.1162175.

6. Ballesteros, Soledad, Julia Mayas, Antonio Prieto, Eloísa Ruiz-Marquez, Pilar Toril, and José M. Reales. 2017. "Effects of Video Game Training on Measures of Selective Attention and Working Memory in Older Adults: Results from a Randomized Controlled Trial." *Frontiers in Aging Neuroscience* 9. doi:10.3389/fnagi.2017.00354.

Chapter 6

1. Vaccaro, Alexandra, Yosef Kaplan Dor, Keishi Nambara, Elizabeth A. Pollina, Cindy Lin, Michael E. Greenberg, and Dragana Rogulja. 2020. "Sleep Loss Can Cause Death through Accumulation of Reactive Oxygen Species in the Gut." *Cell* 181 (6): 1307–1328.e15. doi:10.1016/j.cell.2020.04.049.

2. Reimund, E. 1994. "The Free Radical Flux Theory of Sleep." *Medical Hypotheses* 43 (4): 231–233. doi:10.1016/0306-9877(94)90071-x.

3. Basner, Mathias, Hengyi Rao, Namni Goel, and David F Dinges. 2013. "Sleep Deprivation and Neurobehavioral Dynamics." *Current Opinion in Neurobiology* 23 (5): 854–863. doi:10.1016/j.conb.2013.02.008.

4. You, Jason C., Erica Jones, Devon E. Cross, Abigail C. Lyon, Hyunseung Kang, Andrew B. Newberg, and Carol F. Lippa. 2019. "Association of B-Amyloid Burden with Sleep Dysfunction and Cognitive Impairment in Elderly Individuals with Cognitive Disorders." *JAMA Network Open* 2 (10): e1913383. doi:10.1001/jamanetworkopen.2019.13383.

5. Stepanski, Edward J., and James K. Wyatt. 2003. "Use of Sleep Hygiene in the Treatment of Insomnia." *Sleep Medicine Reviews* 7 (3): 215–225. doi:10.1053/smrv.2001.0246.

6. Riemann, Dieter. 2018. "Sleep Hygiene, Insomnia and Mental Health." *Journal of Sleep Research* 27 (1): 3–3. doi:10.1111/jsr.12661.

7. Rotenberg, Brian W., Dorian Murariu, and Kenny P. Pang. 2016. "Trends in CPAP Adherence over Twenty Years of Data Collection: A Flattened Curve." *Journal of Otolaryngology: Head & Neck Surgery* 45 (1). doi:10.1186/s40463-016-0156-0.

8. Shallcross, Amanda J., Pallavi D. Visvanathan, Sarah H. Sperber, and Zoe T. Duberstein. 2019. "Waking Up to the Problem of Sleep: Can Mindfulness Help? A Review of Theory and Evidence for the Effects of Mindfulness for Sleep." *Current Opinion in Psychology* 28: 37–41. doi:10.1016/j.copsyc.2018.10.005.

9. Fang, Yuan-Yuan, Chia-Tai Hung, Jui-Chun Chan, Sheng-Miauh Huang, and Yun-Hsiang Lee. 2019. "Meta-Analysis: Exercise Intervention for Sleep Problems in Cancer Patients." *European Journal of Cancer Care* 28 (5). doi:10.1111/ecc.13131.

10. Zabrecky, George, Shiva Shahrampour, Cutler Whitely, Mahdi Alizadeh, Chris Conklin, Nancy Wintering, and Karl Doghramji et al. 2020. "An fMRI Study of the Effects of Vibroacoustic Stimulation on Functional Connectivity in Patients with Insomnia." *Sleep Disorders* 2020: 1–9. doi:10.1155/2020/7846914.

Chapter 7

1. Ekman, Paul, and Wallace V. Friesen. 1971. "Constants across Cultures in the Face and Emotion. " *Journal of Personality and Social Psychology* 17 (2): 124–129. doi:10.1037/h0030377.

2. Kontsevich, Leonid L., and Christopher W. Tyler. 2004. "What Makes Mona Lisa Smile?" *Vision Research* 44 (13): 1493–1498. doi:10.1016/j.visres.2003.11.027.

3. Hojat, Mohammadreza, Salvatore Mangione, Thomas Jm Nasca, Susan Rattner, James Bm Erdmann, Joseph Sm Gonnella, and Mike Magee. 2004. "An Empirical Study of Decline in Empathy in Medical School." *Medical Education* 38 (9): 934–941. doi:10.1111/j.1365-2929.2004.01911.x.

4. Holt-Lunstad, Julianne, Timothy B. Smith, and J. Bradley Layton. 2010. "Social Relationships and Mortality Risk: A Meta-Analytic Review." *PloS Medicine* 7 (7): e1000316. doi:10.1371/journal.pmed.1000316.

5. Brooks, David. 2011. *The Social Animal*. New York: Random House.

6. Wintering, Nancy A., Hannah Roggenkamp, Aleezé S. Moss, Judy Shea, Mark R. Waldman, and Andrew Newberg. 2014. "Development and Evaluation of the Belief Acceptance Scale." *Journal of Beliefs & Values* 35 (1): 48–60. doi:10.1080/13617672.2014.884850.

7. Kubota, Jennifer T., Mahzarin R Banaji, and Elizabeth A, Phelps. 2012. "The Neuroscience of Race." *Nature Neuroscience* 15 (7): 940–948. doi:10.1038/nn.3136.

8. Barchas, Denise, Melissa Melaragni, Heather Abrahim, and Eric Barchas. 2020. "The Best Medicine." *Critical Care Nursing Clinics of North America* 32 (2): 167–190. doi:10.1016/j.cnc.2020.01.002; Friedman, E., and C. A. Krause-Parello. 2018. "Companion Animals and Human Health: Benefits, Challenges, and the Road Ahead for Human–Animal Interaction." *Revue Scientifique et Technique de L'oie* 37 (1): 71–82. doi:10.20506/rst.37.1.2741.

Chapter 8

1. Braam, A.W., P. van den Eeden, M. J. Prince, A. T. F. Beekman, S.L. Kivelä, B. A. Lawlor, A. Birkhofer et al. 2001. "Religion as a Cross-Cultural Determinant of Depression in Elderly Europeans: Results from the EURODEP Collaboration." *Psychological Medicine* 31 (5):

803–814. doi:10.1017/s0033291701003956; Koenig, H. G., J. C. Hays, L. K. George, D. G. Blazer, D. B. Larson, & L. R. Landerman. (1997). Modeling the cross-sectional relationships between religion, physical health, social support, and depressive symptoms. *American Journal of Geriatric Psychiatry: Official Journal of the American Association for Geriatric Psychiatry* 5(2), 131–144.

2. Miller, Lisa. 2015. *The Spiritual Child*. New York: St. Martin's Press.

3. Bonelli, Raphael M., and Harold G. Koenig. 2013. "Mental Disorders, Religion and Spirituality 1990 to 2010: A Systematic Evidence-Based Review." *Journal of Religion and Health* 52 (2): 657–673. doi:10.1007/s10943-013-9691-4.

4. Kim, Eric S., Kaitlin A. Hagan, Francine Grodstein, Dawn L. DeMeo, Immaculata De Vivo, and Laura D. Kubzansky. 2016. "Optimism and Cause-Specific Mortality: A Prospective Cohort Study." *American Journal of Epidemiology* 185 (1): 21–29. doi:10.1093/aje/kww182.

5. Newberg, Andrew. 2018. *Neurotheology*. New York: Columbia University Press.

6. Newberg, Andrew B., Eugene G. D'Aquili, and Vince Rause. 2002. *Why God Won't Go Away*. New York: Ballantine Books.

7. Weiner, Gerald A. 2020. "Dark Religion: Fundamentalism from the Perspective of Jungian Psychology. (2018). By Vladislav Solc and George J. Didier. Chiron Publications." *Psychological Perspectives* 63 (2): 304–306. doi:10.1080/00332925.2020.1773169.

8. Monti, Daniel A., Kathryn M. Kash, Elisabeth J. S. Kunkel, George Brainard, Nancy Wintering, Aleezé S. Moss, et al. 2012. "Changes in Cerebral Blood Flow and Anxiety Associated with an 8-Week Mindfulness Programme in Women with Breast Cancer." *Stress and Health* 28 (5): 397–407. doi:10.1002/smi.2470.

9. Moll, J., F. Krueger, R. Zahn, M. Pardini, R. de Oliveira-Souza, and J. Grafman. 2006. "Human Fronto-Mesolimbic Networks Guide Decisions about Charitable Donation." *Proceedings of the National Academy of Sciences* 103 (42): 15623–15628. doi:10.1073/pnas.0604475103.

10. Newberg, Andrew, Michael Pourdehnad, Abass Alavi, and Eugene G. d'Aquili. 2003. "Cerebral Blood Flow during Meditative Prayer: Preliminary Findings and Methodological Issues." *Perceptual and Motor Skills* 97 (2): 625–630. doi:10.2466/pms.2003.97.2.625.

11. Anastasi, Matthew W., and Andrew B. Newberg. 2008. "A Preliminary Study of the Acute Effects of Religious Ritual on Anxiety." *Journal of Alternative and Complementary Medicine* 14 (2): 163–165. doi:10.1089/acm.2007.0675.

12. Newberg, Andrew B., Nancy A. Wintering, Donna Morgan, and Mark R. Waldman. 2006. "The Measurement of Regional Cerebral Blood Flow during Glossolalia: A Preliminary SPECT Study." *Psychiatry Research: Neuroimaging* 148 (1): 67–71. doi:10.1016/j.pscychresns.2006.07.001.

Chapter 9

1. Barnes, Jill N., and Adam T. Corkery. 2018. "Exercise Improves Vascular Function, But Does This Translate to the Brain?" *Brain Plasticity* 4 (1): 65–79. doi:10.3233/bpl-180075.

2. Rivest-Gadbois, Emmanuelle, and Marie-Hélène Boudrias. 2019. "What Are the Known Effects of Yoga on the Brain in Relation to Motor Performances, Body Awareness and Pain? A Narrative Review." *Complementary Therapies in Medicine* 44: 129–142. doi:10.1016/j.ctim.2019.03.021.

3. Mooventhan, A., and L. Nivethitha. 2017. "Evidence Based Effects of Yoga in Neurological Disorders." *Journal of Clinical Neuroscience* 43: 61–67. doi:10.1016/j.jocn.2017.05.012.

4. Mahalakshmi, B., Nancy Maurya, Shin-Da Lee, and V. Bharath Kumar. 2020. "Possible Neuroprotective Mechanisms of Physical Exercise in Neurodegeneration." *International Journal of Molecular Sciences* 21 (16): 5895. doi:10.3390/ijms21165895.

5. Best, John R., Bryan K. Chiu, Peter A. Hall, and Teresa Liu-Ambrose. 2017. "Larger Lateral Prefrontal Cortex Volume Predicts Better Exercise Adherence among Older Women: Evidence from Two Exercise Training Studies." *Journals of Gerontology: Series A* 72 (6): 804–810. doi:10.1093/gerona/glx043.

6. Azevedo, Kesley Pablo Morais de, Victor Hugo de Oliveira, Gidyenne Christine Bandeira Silva de Medeiros, Ádala Nayana de Sousa Mata, Daniel Ángel García, Daniel Guillén Martínez, et al. 2020. "The Effects of Exercise on BDNF Levels in Adolescents: A Systematic Review with Meta-Analysis." *International Journal of Environmental Research and Public Health* 17 (17): 6056. doi:10.3390/ijerph17176056.

7. Meeusen, Romain, and Kenny De Meirleir. 1995. "Exercise and Brain Neurotransmission." *Sports Medicine* 20 (3): 160–188. doi:10.2165/00007256-199520030-00004.

Chapter 10

1. Lupien, Sonia J., Bruce S. McEwen, Megan R. Gunnar, and Christine Heim. 2009. "Effects of Stress throughout the Lifespan on the Brain, Behaviour and Cognition." *Nature Reviews Neuroscience* 10 (6): 434–445. doi:10.1038/nrn2639.

2. Kunimatsu, Akira, Koichiro Yasaka, Hiroyuki Akai, Natsuko Kunimatsu, and Osamu Abe. 2019. "MRI Findings in Posttraumatic Stress Disorder." *Journal of Magnetic Resonance Imaging* 52 (2): 380–396. doi:10.1002/jmri.26929.

3. Kabat-Zinn, Jon. 1990. *Full Catastrophe Living.* New York: Delacorte Press.

4. Monti, Daniel A., Anna Tobia, Marie Stoner, Nancy Wintering, Michael Matthews, Xiao-Song He, et al. 2017. "Neuro Emotional Technique Effects on Brain Physiology in Cancer Patients with Traumatic Stress Symptoms: Preliminary Findings." *Journal of Cancer Survivorship* 11 (4): 438–446. doi:10.1007/s11764-017-0601-8.

5. Newberg, Andrew B., Nancy Wintering, Dharma S. Khalsa, Hannah Roggenkamp, and Mark R. Waldman. 2010. "Meditation Effects on Cognitive Function and Cerebral Blood Flow in Subjects with Memory Loss: A Preliminary Study." *Journal of Alzheimer's Disease* 20 (2): 517–526. doi:10.3233/jad-2010-1391.

6. Moss, Aleezé Sattar, Nancy Wintering, Hannah Roggenkamp, Dharma Singh Khalsa, Mark R. Waldman, Daniel Monti, and Andrew B. Newberg. 2012. "Effects of an 8-Week Meditation Program on Mood and Anxiety in Patients with Memory Loss." *Journal of Alternative and Complementary Medicine* 18 (1): 48–53. doi:10.1089/acm.2011.0051.

7. F. Masana, Maria, Stefanos Tyrovolas, Natasa Kollia, Christina Chrysohoou, John Skoumas, Josep Maria Haro, et al. 2019. "Dietary Patterns and Their Association with Anxiety Symptoms among Older Adults: the ATTICA Study." *Nutrients* 11 (6): 1250. doi:10.3390/nu11061250.

8. Gibson-Smith, D., M. Bot, I. Brouwer, M. Visser, and B. W. J. H. Penninx. 2018. "Diet Quality in Subjects with and without Depressive and Anxiety Disorders." *Proceedings of the Nutrition Society* 77 (OCE2). doi:10.1017/s0029665118000332.

9. "Gamma-aminobutyric acid (GABA), Monograph." 2007. *Alternative Medicine Review: A Journal of Clinical Therapeutic* 12 (3): 274–9.

10. Williams, Jackson L., Julian M. Everett, Nathan M. D'Cunha, Domenico Sergi, Ekavi N. Georgousopoulou, Richard J. Keegan, et al. 2019. "The Effects of Green Tea Amino Acid L-Theanine Consumption on the Ability to Manage Stress and Anxiety Levels: A Systematic Review." *Plant Foods for Human Nutrition* 75 (1): 12–23. doi:10.1007/s11130-019-00771-5.

11. Lopresti, Adrian L., Stephen J. Smith, Hakeemudin Malvi, and Rahul Kodgule. 2019. "An Investigation into the Stress-Relieving and Pharmacological Actions of An Ashwagandha (Withania somnifera) Extract." *Medicine* 98 (37): e17186. doi:10.1097/md.0000000000017186.

12. Calabrese, Carlo, William L. Gregory, Michael Leo, Dale Kraemer, Kerry Bone, and Barry Oken. 2008. "Effects of a Standardized Bacopa Monnieri Extract on Cognitive Performance, Anxiety, and Depression in the Elderly: A Randomized, Double-Blind, Placebo-Controlled Trial." *Journal of Alternative and Complementary Medicine* 14 (6): 707–713. doi:10.1089/acm.2008.0018.

13. Farshbaf-Khalili, Azizeh, Mahin Kamalifard, and Mahsa Namadian. 2018. "Comparison of the Effect of Lavender and Bitter Orange on Anxiety in Postmenopausal Women: A Triple-Blind, Randomized, Controlled Clinical Trial." *Complementary Therapies in Clinical Practice* 31: 132–138. doi:10.1016/j.ctcp.2018.02.004.

14. Zamanifar, Somayeh, Mohammad Iraj Bagheri-Saveh, A. Nezakati, Rozhin Mohammadi, and J. Seidi. "The Effect of Music Therapy and Aromatherapy with Chamomile-Lavender Essential Oil on the Anxiety of Clinical Nurses: A Randomized and Double-Blind Clinical Trial." *Journal of Medicine and Life* 13 (2020): 87–93.

15. Akhondzadeh, S., H. R. Naghavi, M. Vazirian, A. Shayeganpour, H. Rashidi, and M. Khani. 2001. "Passionflower in the Treatment of Generalized Anxiety: A Pilot Double-Blind Randomized Controlled Trial with Oxazepam." *Journal of Clinical Pharmacy and Therapeutics* 26 (5): 363–367. doi:10.1046/j.1365-2710.2001.00367.x.

16. Cropley, Mark, Adrian P. Banks, and Julia Boyle. 2015. "The Effects Of Rhodiola rosea L. Extract on Anxiety, Stress, Cognition and Other Mood Symptoms." *Phytotherapy Research* 29 (12): 1934–1939. doi:10.1002/ptr.5486.

Chapter 11

1. Monti, Daniel A., Kathryn M. Kash, Elisabeth J. S. Kunkel, George Brainard, Nancy Wintering, Aleezé S. Moss, et al. 2012. "Changes in Cerebral Blood Flow and Anxiety Associated with an 8-Week Mindfulness Programme in Women with Breast Cancer." *Stress and Health* 28 (5): 397–407. doi:10.1002/smi.2470.

2. De Pisapia, Nicola, Francesca Bacci, Danielle Parrott, and David Melcher. 2016. "Brain Networks for Visual Creativity: A Functional Connectivity Study of Planning a Visual Artwork." *Scientific Reports* 6 (1). doi:10.1038/srep39185.

3. Bubna, Ketan, Sapna Hegde, and Dinesh Rao. 2017. "Role of Colors in Pediatric Dental Practices." *Journal of Clinical Pediatric Dentistry* 41 (3): 193–198. doi:10.17796/1053-4628-41.3.193.

4. Ayoub, Chakib M., Laudi B. Rizk, Chadi I. Yaacoub, Dorothy Gaal, and Zeev N. Kain. 2005. "Music and Ambient Operating Room Noise in Patients Undergoing Spinal Anesthesia." *Anesthesia & Analgesia* 100 (5): 1316–1319. doi:10.1213/01.ane.0000153014.46893.9b; Ullmann, Yehuda, Lucian Fodor, Irena Schwarzberg, Nurit Carmi, Amos Ullmann, and Yitzchak Ramon. 2008. "The Sounds of Music in the Operating Room." *Injury* 39 (5): 592–597. doi:10.1016/j.injury.2006.06.021.

5. Newberg, Andrew B., Nancy Wintering, Dharma S. Khalsa, Hannah Roggenkamp, and Mark R. Waldman. 2010. "Meditation Effects on Cognitive Function and Cerebral Blood Flow in Subjects with Memory Loss: A Preliminary Study." *Journal of Alzheimer's Disease* 20 (2): 517–526. doi:10.3233/jad-2010-1391.

6. Chrysikou, Evangelia G., Christopher Wertz, David B. Yaden, Scott Barry Kaufman, Donna Bacon, Nancy A. Wintering, et al. 2020. "Differences in Brain Morphometry Associated with Creative Performance in High- and Average-Creative Achievers." *Neuroimage* 218: 116921. doi:10.1016/j.neuroimage.2020.116921; Chrysikou, Evangelia G., Constanza Jacial, David B. Yaden, Wessel van Dam, Scott Barry Kaufman, Christopher J. Conklin, et al. 2020. "Differences in Brain Activity Patterns during Creative Idea Generation between Eminent and Non-Eminent Thinkers." *Neuroimage* 220: 117011. doi:10.1016/j.neuroimage.2020.117011.

Chapter 12

1. Nash, Jonathan D., Andrew Newberg, and Bhuvanesh Awasthi. 2019. "Corrigendum: Toward a Unifying Taxonomy and Definition for Meditation." *Frontiers in Psychology* 10. doi:10.3389/fpsyg.2019.02206.

2. Johnson, Kyle D., Hengyi Rao, Nancy Wintering, Namisha Dhillon, Siyuan Hu, Senhua Zhu, Marc Korczykowski, et al. 2014. "Pilot Study of the Effect of Religious Symbols on Brain Function: Association with Measures of Religiosity." *Spirituality in Clinical Practice* 1 (2): 82–98. doi:10.1037/scp0000015.

3. Newberg, Andrew B., Nancy Wintering, Dharma S. Khalsa, Hannah Roggenkamp, and Mark R. Waldman. 2010. "Meditation Effects on Cognitive Function and Cerebral Blood Flow in Subjects with Memory Loss: A Preliminary Study." *Journal of Alzheimer's Disease* 20 (2): 517–526. doi:10.3233/jad-2010-1391.

4. Hofmann, Stefan G., and Angelina F. Gómez. 2017. "Mindfulness-Based Interventions for Anxiety and Depression." *Psychiatric Clinics of North America* 40 (4): 739–749. doi:10.1016/j.psc.2017.08.008.

5. Cohen, Debbie L., Nancy Wintering, Victoria Tolles, Raymond R. Townsend, John T. Farrar, Mary Lou Galantino, and Andrew B. Newberg. 2009. "Cerebral Blood Flow Effects of Yoga Training: Preliminary Evaluation of 4 Cases." *Journal of Alternative and Complementary Medicine* 15 (1): 9–14. doi:10.1089/acm.2008.0008.

6. Brinsley, Jacinta, Felipe Schuch, Oscar Lederman, Danielle Girard, Matthew Smout, Maarten A. Immink et al. 2020. "Effects of Yoga on Depressive Symptoms in People with Mental Disorders: A Systematic Review and Meta-Analysis." *British Journal of Sports Medicine*, bjsports-2019-101242. doi:10.1136/bjsports-2019-101242.

7. Blake, Holly, and Helen Hawley. 2012. "Effects of Tai Chi Exercise on Physical and Psychological Health of Older People." *Current Aging Science* 5 (1): 19–27. doi:10.2174/1874609811205010019.

Chapter 13

1. Elkins, Gary R., Arreed F. Barabasz, James R. Council, and David Spiegel. 2015. "Advancing Research and Practice: The Revised APA Division 30 Definition of Hypnosis." *American Journal of Clinical Hypnosis* 57 (4): 378–385. doi:10.1080/00029157.2015.1011465.

2. Cojan, Yann, Camille Piguet, and Patrik Vuilleumier. 2015. "What Makes Your Brain Suggestible? Hypnotizability Is Associated with Differential Brain Activity during Attention Outside Hypnosis." *Neuroimage* 117: 367–374. doi:10.1016/j.neuroimage.2015.05.076.

3. Heunis, Stephan, Rolf Lamerichs, Svitlana Zinger, Cesar Caballero-Gaudes, Jacobus F. A. Jansen, Bert Aldenkamp, and Marcel Breeuwer. 2020. "Quality and Denoising in Real-Time Functional Magnetic Resonance Imaging Neurofeedback: A Methods Review." *Human Brain Mapping* 41 (12): 3439–3467. doi:10.1002/hbm.25010.

4. Monti, Daniel A., Anna Tobia, Marie Stoner, Nancy Wintering, Michael Matthews, Chris J. Conklin et al. 2017. "Changes in Cerebellar Functional Connectivity and Autonomic Regulation in Cancer Patients Treated with the Neuro Emotional Technique for Traumatic Stress Symptoms." *Journal of Cancer Survivorship* 12 (1): 145–153. doi:10.1007/s11764-017-0653-9; Monti, Daniel A., Anna Tobia, Marie Stoner, Nancy Wintering, Michael Matthews, Xiao-Song He et al. 2017. "Neuro Emotional Technique Effects on Brain Physiology in Cancer Patients with Traumatic Stress Symptoms: Preliminary Findings." *Journal of Cancer Survivorship* 11 (4): 438–446. doi:10.1007/s11764-017-0601-8.

5. Dossett, Michelle, and Gloria Yeh. 2017. "Homeopathy Use in the United States and Implications for Public Health: A Review." *Homeopathy* 107 (01): 003-009. doi:10.1055/s-0037-1609016.

6. Linde, Klaus, Nicola Clausius, Gilbert Ramirez, Dieter Melchart, Florian Eitel, Larry V Hedges, and Wayne B Jonas. "Are the Clinical Effects of Homeopathy Placebo Effects? A Meta-Analysis of Placebo-Controlled Trials." *The Lancet* 350, no. 9081 (1997): 834–843. doi:10.1016/s0140-6736(97)02293-9.

7. Banerjee S, Argaez C. "Eye Movement Desensitization and Reprocessing for Depression, Anxiety, and Post-Traumatic Stress Disorder: A Review of Clinical Effectiveness" [Internet]. Ottawa (ON): Canadian Agency for Drugs and Technologies in Health; 2017. PMID:30160866. 2021.

8. Stein, Dirson João, Liciane Fernandes Medeiros, Wolnei Caumo, and Iraci LS Torres. 2020. "Transcranial Direct Current Stimulation in Patients with Anxiety: Current Perspectives." *Neuropsychiatric Disease and Treatment* 16: 161–169. doi:10.2147/ndt.s195840; Moffa, Adriano H., Donel Martin, Angelo Alonzo, Djamila Bennabi, Daniel M. Blumberger, Isabela M. Benseñor, Zafiris Daskalakis et al. 2020. "Efficacy and Acceptability of Transcranial Direct Current Stimulation (tDCS) for Major Depressive Disorder: An Individual Patient Data Meta-Analysis." *Progress in Neuro-Psychopharmacology and Biological Psychiatry* 99: 109836. doi:10.1016/j.pnpbp.2019.109836.

9. da Silva, Morgana Croce, Catarine Lima Conti, Jaisa Klauss, Luana Gaburro Alves, Henrique Mineiro do Nascimento Cavalcante, Felipe Fregni, et al. 2013. "Behavioral Effects of Transcranial Direct Current Stimulation (TDCS) Induced Dorsolateral Prefrontal Cortex Plasticity in Alcohol Dependence." *Journal of Physiology–Paris* 107 (6): 493–502. doi:10.1016/j.jphysparis.2013.07.003.

Chapter 14

1. Lewis, Glyn. 1996. "DSM-IV. Diagnostic and Statistical Manual of Mental Disorders, 4th Edition by the American Psychiatric Association. (Pp. 886; £34.95.) APA: Washington, DC.1994." *Psychological Medicine* 26 (3): 651–652. doi:10.1017/s0033291700035765.

2. Carmassi, Claudia, Claudia Foghi, Valerio Dell'Oste, Carlo Antonio Bertelloni, Andrea Fiorillo, and Liliana Dell'Osso. 2020. "Risk and Protective Factors for PTSD in Caregivers of Adult Patients with Severe Medical Illnesses: A Systematic Review." *International Journal of Environmental Research and Public Health* 17 (16): 5888. doi:10.3390/ijerph17165888.

3. Lange, Iris, Zuzana Kasanova, Liesbet Goossens, Nicole Leibold, Chris I. De Zeeuw, Therese van Amelsvoort, and Koen Schruers. 2015. "The Anatomy of Fear Learning in the Cerebellum: A Systematic Meta-Analysis." *Neuroscience & Biobehavioral Reviews* 59: 83–91. doi:10.1016/j.neubiorev.2015.09.019; Öhman, Arne. 2005. "The Role of the Amygdala in Human Fear: Automatic Detection of Threat." *Psychoneuroendocrinology* 30 (10): 953–958. doi:10.1016/j.psyneuen.2005.03.019.

4. Nutt, David J., James C. Ballenger, David Sheehan, and Hans-Ulrich Wittchen. 2002. "Generalized Anxiety Disorder: Comorbidity, Comparative Biology and Treatment." *International Journal of Neuropsychopharmacology* 5 (4): 315–325. doi:10.1017/s1461145702003048.

5. Goddard, Andrew W., Graeme F. Mason, Ahmad Almai, Douglas L. Rothman, Kevin L. Behar, Ognen A. C. Petroff, et al. 2001. "Reductions in Occipital Cortex GABA Levels in Panic Disorder Detected with 1H-Magnetic Resonance Spectroscopy." *Archives of General Psychiatry* 58 (6): 556. doi:10.1001/archpsyc.58.6.556.

6. Jacka, Felice N., Julie A. Pasco, Arnstein Mykletun, Lana J. Williams, Allison M. Hodge, Sharleen Linette O'Reilly, et al. 2010. "Association of Western and Traditional Diets with Depression and Anxiety in Women." *American Journal of Psychiatry* 167 (3): 305–311. doi:10.1176/appi.ajp.2009.09060881.

7. Jacka, Felice N., Arnstein Mykletun, Michael Berk, Ingvar Bjelland, and Grethe S. Tell. 2011. "The Association between Habitual Diet Quality and the Common Mental Disorders in Community-Dwelling Adults." *Psychosomatic Medicine* 73 (6): 483–490. doi:10.1097/psy.0b013e318222831a.

8. Robert P. Hoffman. 2007. "Sympathetic Mechanisms of Hypoglycemic Counterregulation." *Current Diabetes Reviews* 3 (3): 185–193. doi:10.2174/157339907781368995.

9. Maqsood, Raeesah, and Trevor W. Stone. 2016. "The Gut-Brain Axis, BDNF, NMDA and CNS Disorders." *Neurochemical Research* 41 (11): 2819–2835. doi:10.1007/s11064-016-2039-1.

10. Sarris, J., S. Moylan, D. A. Camfield, M. P. Pase, D. Mischoulon, M. Berk, F. N. Jacka, and I. Schweitzer. 2012. "Complementary Medicine, Exercise, Meditation, Diet, and Lifestyle Modification for Anxiety Disorders: A Review of Current Evidence." *Evidence-Based Complementary and Alternative Medicine* 2012: 1–20. doi:10.1155/2012/809653.

11. Deslandes, Andréa, Helena Moraes, Camila Ferreira, Heloisa Veiga, Heitor Silveira, Raphael Mouta, Fernando A.M.S. Pompeu, et al. 2009. "Exercise and Mental Health: Many Reasons to Move." *Neuropsychobiology* 59 (4): 191–198. doi:10.1159/000223730.

12. Wipfli, Bradley M., Chad D. Rethorst, and Daniel M. Landers. 2008. "The Anxiolytic Effects of Exercise: A Meta-Analysis of Randomized Trials and Dose–Response Analysis." *Journal of Sport and Exercise Psychology* 30 (4): 392–410. doi:10.1123/jsep.30.4.392.

13. Hofmann, Stefan G., Alice T. Sawyer, Ashley A. Witt, and Diana Oh. 2010. "The Effect of Mindfulness-Based Therapy on Anxiety and Depression: A Meta-Analytic Review." *Journal of Consulting and Clinical Psychology* 78 (2): 169–183. doi:10.1037/a0018555.

14. Newberg, Andrew B., Nancy Wintering, David B. Yaden, Li Zhong, Brendan Bowen, Noah Averick, and Daniel A. Monti. 2017. "Effect of a One-Week Spiritual Retreat on Dopamine and Serotonin Transporter Binding: A Preliminary Study." *Religion, Brain & Behavior* 8 (3): 265–278. doi:10.1080/2153599x.2016.1267035.

15. Webster, Craig S., Anna Y. Luo, Chris Krägeloh, Fiona Moir, and Marcus Henning. 2016. "A Systematic Review of the Health Benefits of Tai Chi for Students in Higher Education." *Preventive Medicine Reports* 3: 103–112. doi:10.1016/j.pmedr.2015.12.006.

16. Mofredj, A., S. Alaya, K. Tassaioust, H. Bahloul, and A. Mrabet. 2016. "Music Therapy: A Review of the Potential Therapeutic Benefits for the Critically Ill." *Journal of Critical Care* 35: 195–199. doi:10.1016/j.jcrc.2016.05.021.

17. Bradt, Joke, and Cheryl Dileo. 2014. "Music Interventions for Mechanically Ventilated Patients." *Cochrane Database of Systematic Reviews.* doi:10.1002/14651858.cd006902.pub3.

18. Monti, Daniel A., Caroline Peterson, Elisabeth J. Shakin Kunkel, Walter W. Hauck, Edward Pequignot, Lora Rhodes, and George C. Brainard. 2006. "A Randomized, Controlled Trial of Mindfulness-Based Art Therapy (MBAT) for Women with Cancer." *Psycho-Oncology* 15 (5): 363–373. doi:10.1002/pon.988; Eum, Yeongcheol, and Jongeun Yim. 2015. "Literature and Art Therapy in Post-Stroke Psychological Disorders." *Tohoku Journal of Experimental Medicine* 235 (1): 17–23. doi:10.1620/tjem.235.17.

19. Black, Shaun, Kathleen Jacques, Adam Webber, Kathy Spurr, Eileen Carey, Andrea Hebb, and Robert Gilbert. 2010. "Chair Massage for Treating Anxiety in Patients Withdrawing from Psychoactive Drugs." *Journal of Alternative and Complementary Medicine* 16 (9): 979–987. doi:10.1089/acm.2009.0645.

20. Black, Shaun, Kathleen Jacques, Adam Webber, Kathy Spurr, Eileen Carey, Andrea Hebb, and Robert Gilbert. 2010. "Chair Massage for Treating Anxiety in Patients Withdrawing from Psychoactive Drugs." *Journal of Alternative and Complementary Medicine* 16 (9): 979–987. doi:10.1089/acm.2009.0645.

21. Baldwin, David S., and Claire Polkinghorn. 2005. "Evidence-Based Pharmacotherapy of Generalized Anxiety Disorder." *International Journal of Neuropsychopharmacology* 8 (2): 293–302. doi:10.1017/s1461145704004870.

22. Evans, Susan, Stephen Ferrando, Marianne Findler, Charles Stowell, Colette Smart, and Dean Haglin. 2008. "Mindfulness-Based Cognitive Therapy for Generalized Anxiety Disorder." *Journal of Anxiety Disorders* 22 (4): 716–721. doi:10.1016/j.janxdis.2007.07.005.

23. "Cognitive-Behavioral Therapy for Anxiety Disorders: An Update on the Empirical Evidence." 2015. *Anxiety* 17 (3): 337–346. doi:10.31887/dcns.2015.17.3/akaczkurkin.

24. Salzer, Simone, Christel Winkelbach, Frank Leweke, Eric Leibing, and Falk Leichsenring. 2011. "Long-Term Effects of Short-Term Psychodynamic Psychotherapy and Cognitive-Behavioural Therapy in Generalized Anxiety Disorder: 12-Month Follow–Up." *Canadian Journal of Psychiatry* 56 (8): 503–508. doi:10.1177/070674371105600809.

25. Ellis, Albert. 2003. "Early Theories and Practices of Rational Emotive Behavior Therapy and How They Have Been Augmented and Revised during the Last Three Decades." *Journal of Rational-Emotive and Cognitive-Behavior Therapy* 21 (3/4): 219–243. doi:10.1023/a:1025890112319.

26. Hanus, Michel, Jacqueline Lafon, and Marc Mathieu. 2003. "Double-Blind, Randomised, Placebo-Controlled Study to Evaluate the Efficacy and Safety of a Fixed Combination Containing Two Plant Extracts (Crataegus oxyacantha and Eschscholtzia californica) and Magnesium in Mild-to-Moderate Anxiety Disorders." *Current Medical Research and Opinion* 20 (1): 63–71. doi:10.1185/030079903125002603.

27. Kasper, Siegfried, Markus Gastpar, Walter E. Müller, Hans-Peter Volz, Hans-Jürgen Möller, Angelika Dienel, and Sandra Schläfke. 2010. "Silexan, An Orally Administered Lavandula Oil Preparation, Is Effective in the Treatment of 'Subsyndromal' Anxiety Disorder:

A Randomized, Double-Blind, Placebo Controlled Trial." *International Clinical Psychopharmacology* 25 (5): 277–287. doi:10.1097/yic.0b013e32833b3242.

28. Kasper, Siegfried, Markus Gastpar, Walter E. Müller, Hans-Peter Volz, Hans-Jürgen Möller, Angelika Dienel, and Sandra Schläfke. 2010. "Silexan, an Orally Administered Lavandula Oil Preparation, Is Effective in the Treatment of 'Subsyndromal' Anxiety Disorder: A Randomized, Double-Blind, Placebo Controlled Trial." *International Clinical Psychopharmacology* 25 (5): 277–287. doi:10.1097/yic.0b013e32833b3242.

29. Kennedy, David O., Wendy Little, and Andrew B. Scholey. 2004. "Attenuation of Laboratory-Induced Stress in Humans After Acute Administration of Melissa officinalis (Lemon Balm)." *Psychosomatic Medicine* 66 (4): 607–613. doi:10.1097/01.psy.0000132877.72833.71.

30. Mao, Jun J., Sharon X. Xie, John R. Keefe, Irene Soeller, Qing S. Li, and Jay D. Amsterdam. 2016. "Long–Term Chamomile (Matricaria chamomilla L.) Treatment for Generalized Anxiety Disorder: A Randomized Clinical Trial." *Phytomedicine* 23 (14): 1735–1742. doi:10.1016/j.phymed.2016.10.012.

31. Pittler, Max H., and Edzard Ernst. 2003. „Kava Extract Versus Placebo for Treating Anxiety." *Cochrane Database of Systematic Reviews*. doi:10.1002/14651858.cd003383.

32. Vargas, Ana Sofia, Ângelo Luís, Mário Barroso, Eugenia Gallardo, and Luísa Pereira. 2020. "Psilocybin As A New Approach to Treat Depression and Anxiety in the Context of Life-Threatening Diseases—A Systematic Review and Meta-Analysis of Clinical Trials." *Biomedicines* 8 (9): 331. doi:10.3390/biomedicines8090331.

Chapter 15

1. Kumar, A., A. Newberg, A. Alavi, J. Berlin, R. Smith, and M. Reivich. 1993. "Regional Cerebral Glucose Metabolism in Late-Life Depression and Alzheimer Disease: A Preliminary Positron Emission Tomography Study." *Proceedings of the National Academy of Sciences* 90 (15): 7019–7023. doi:10.1073/pnas.90.15.7019.

2. Hryhorczuk, Cecile, Sandeep Sharma, and Stephanie E. Fulton. 2013. "Metabolic Disturbances Connecting Obesity and Depression." *Frontiers in Neuroscience* 7. doi:10.3389/fnins.2013.00177.

3. Brenes, G. A., J. D. Williamson, S. P. Messier, W. J. Rejeski, M. Pahor, E. Ip, and B. W. J. H. Penninx. 2007. "Treatment of Minor Depression in Older Adults: A Pilot Study Comparing Sertraline and Exercise." *Aging & Mental Health* 11 (1): 61–68. doi:10.1080/13607860600736372;11(1):61–8; Blumenthal, James A., Michael A. Babyak, P Murali Doraiswamy, Lana Watkins, Benson M. Hoffman, Krista A. Barbour, and Steve Herman et al. 2007. "Exercise and Pharmacotherapy in the Treatment of Major Depressive Disorder." *Psychosomatic Medicine* 69 (7): 587–596. doi:10.1097/psy.0b013e318148c19a.

4. Knubben, K., F. M. Reischies, M. Adli, P. Schlattmann, M. Bauer, F. Dimeo, and L. Ansley. 2006. "A Randomised, Controlled Study on the Effects of a Short-Term Endurance Training Programme in Patients with Major Depression Commentary." *British Journal of Sports Medicine* 41 (1): 29–33. doi:10.1136/bjsm.2006.030130; Trivedi, Madhukar H., Tracy L. Greer, Bruce D. Grannemann, Heather O. Chambliss, and Alexander N. Jordan. 2006. "Exercise as an Augmentation Strategy for Treatment of Major Depression." *Journal of Psychiatric Practice* 12 (4): 205–213. doi:10.1097/00131746-200607000-00002.

5. Kamei, Tsutomu, Yoshitaka Toriumi, Hiroshi Kimura, Hiroaki Kumano, Satoshi Ohno, and Keishin Kimura. 2000. "Decrease in Serum Cortisol during Yoga Exercise Is Correlated with Alpha Wave Activation." *Perceptual and Motor Skills* 90 (3): 1027–1032. doi:10.2466/pms.2000.90.3.1027.

6. Braam, A. W., A. T. F. Beekman, D. J. H. Deeg, J. H. Smit, and W. Tilburg. 1997. "Religiosity as a Protective or Prognostic Factor of Depression in Later Life: Results from a Community Survey in the Netherlands." *Acta Psychiatrica Scandinavica* 96 (3): 199–205. doi:10.1111/j.1600-0447.1997.tb10152.x.

7. Miller, Lisa. 2015. *The Spiritual Child.* New York: St. Martin's Press.

8. Freeman, Marlene P., Maurizio Fava, James Lake, Madhukar H. Trivedi, Katherine L. Wisner, and David Mischoulon. 2010. "Complementary and Alternative Medicine in Major Depressive Disorder." *Journal of Clinical Psychiatry* 71 (6): 669–681. doi:10.4088/jcp.10cs05959blu.

9. Linde, K., and L. Knüppel. 2005. "Large-Scale Observational Studies of Hypericum Extracts in Patients with Depressive Disorders—A Systematic Review." *Phytomedicine* 12 (1–2): 148–157. doi:10.1016/j.phymed.2004.02.004.

10. Gurley, Bill J., Ashley Swain, D. Keith Williams, Gary Barone, and Sunil K. Battu. 2008. "Gauging the Clinical Significance of P-Glycoprotein-Mediated Herb-Drug Interactions: Comparative Effects of St. John's Wort, Echinacea, Clarithromycin, and Rifampin on Digoxin Pharmacokinetics." *Molecular Nutrition & Food Research* 52 (7): 772–779. doi:10.1002/mnfr.200700081.

11. Moses, Eydie L., and Alan G. Mallinger. 2000. "St. John's Wort: Three Cases of Possible Mania Induction." *Journal of Clinical Psychopharmacology* 20 (1): 115–117. doi:10.1097/00004714-200002000-00027.

12. Boyer, Edward W., and Michael Shannon. 2005. "The Serotonin Syndrome." *New England Journal of Medicine* 352 (11): 1112–1120. doi:10.1056/nejmra041867.

13. Chouinard, Guy, Linda Beauclair, Rita Geiser, and Pierre Etienne. 1990. "A Pilot Study of Magnesium Aspartate Hydrochloride (Magnesiocard) as a Mood Stabilizer for Rapid Cycling Bipolar Affective Disorder Patients." *Progress in Neuro-Psychopharmacology and Biological Psychiatry* 14 (2): 171–180. doi:10.1016/0278-5846(90)90099-3.

14. Heiden, Angela, Richard Frey, Otto Presslich, Thomas Blasbichler, Ronald Smetana, and Siegfried Kasper. 1999. "Treatment of Severe Mania with Intravenous Magnesium Sulphate as a Supplementary Therapy." *Psychiatry Research* 89 (3): 239–246. doi:10.1016/s0165-1781(99)00107-9.

15. Chengappa, Kn Roy, Joseph Levine, Samuel Gershon, Alan G Mallinger, Antonio Hardan, Anthony Vagnucci, and Bruce Pollock et al. 2000. "Inositol as an Add-On Treatment for Bipolar Depression." *Bipolar Disorders* 2 (1): 47–55. doi:10.1034/j.1399-5618.2000.020107.x; Eden Evins, A., Christina Demopulos, Iftah Yovel, Melissa Culhane, Jacqueline Ogutha, Louisa D. Grandin, et al. 2006. "Inositol Augmentation of Lithium or Valproate for Bipolar Depression." *Bipolar Disorders* 8 (2): 168–174. doi:10.1111/j.1399-5618.2006.00303.x.

16. Bell, Iris R., Joel S. Edman, David W. Marby, Andrew Satlin, Theodore Dreier, Benjamin Liptzin, and Jonathan O. Cole. 1990. "Vitamin B12 and Folate Status in Acute Geropsychiatric Inpatients: Affective and Cognitive Characteristics of a Vitamin Nondeficient Population." *Biological Psychiatry* 27 (2): 125–137. doi:10.1016/0006-3223(90)90642-f.

17. Dyall, S. C., and A. T. Michael-Titus. 2008. "Neurological Benefits of Omega-3 Fatty Acids." *Neuromolecular Medicine* 10 (4): 219–235. doi:10.1007/s12017-008-8036-z.

18. Stoll, Andrew L., W. Emanuel Severus, Marlene P. Freeman, Stephanie Rueter, Holly A. Zboyan, Eli Diamond, et al. 1999. "Omega 3 Fatty Acids in Bipolar Disorder." *Archives of General Psychiatry* 56 (5): 407. doi:10.1001/archpsyc.56.5.407.

19. Osher, Yamima, Yuly Bersudsky, and R. H. Belmaker. 2005. "Omega-3 Eicosapentaenoic Acid in Bipolar Depression." *Journal of Clinical Psychiatry* 66 (6): 726–729. doi:10.4088/jcp.v66n0608.

20. Frangou, Sophia, Michael Lewis, and Paul McCrone. 2006. "Efficacy of Ethyl-Eicosapentaenoic Acid in Bipolar Depression: Randomised Double-Blind Placebo-Controlled Study." *British Journal of Psychiatry* 188 (1): 46–50. doi:10.1192/bjp.188.1.46.

21. Hirashima, Fuyuki, Aimee M. Parow, Andrew L. Stoll, Christina M. Demopulos, Karen E. Damico, Michael L. Rohan, Justin G. Eskesen, Chun S. Zuo, Bruce M. Cohen, and Perry F. Renshaw. 2004. "Omega-3 Fatty Acid Treatment and T2 Whole Brain Relaxation Times in Bipolar Disorder." *American Journal of Psychiatry* 161 (10): 1922–1924. doi:10.1176/ajp.161.10.1922.

22. Sarris, Jerome, James Lake, and Rogier Hoenders. 2011. „Bipolar Disorder and Complementary Medicine: Current Evidence, Safety Issues, and Clinical Considerations." *Journal of Alternative and Complementary Medicine* 17 (10): 881–890. doi:10.1089/acm.2010.0481.

23. Scarnà, A., H. J. Gijsman, S. F. B. Mctavish, C. J. Harmer, P. J. Cowen, and G. M. Goodwin. 2003. "Effects of a Branched-Chain Amino Acid Drink in Mania." *British Journal of Psychiatry* 182 (3): 210–213. doi:10.1192/bjp.182.3.210.

24. Berk, Michael, David L. Copolov, Olivia Dean, Kristy Lu, Sue Jeavons, Ian Schapkaitz, et al. 2008. "N-Acetyl Cysteine for Depressive Symptoms in Bipolar Disorder—A Double-Blind Randomized Placebo-Controlled Trial." *Biological Psychiatry* 64 (6): 468–475. doi:10.1016/j.biopsych.2008.04.022.

25. Sarris, Jerome, David Mischoulon, and Isaac Schweitzer. 2011. „Adjunctive Nutraceuticals with Standard Pharmacotherapies in Bipolar Disorder: A Systematic Review of Clinical Trials." *Bipolar Disorders* 13 (5–6): 454–465. doi:10.1111/j.1399-5618.2011.00945.x.

26. Moses, Eydie L., and Alan G. Mallinger. 2000. "St. John's Wort: Three Cases of Possible Mania Induction." *Journal of Clinical Psychopharmacology* 20 (1): 115–117. doi:10.1097/00004714-200002000-00027.

27. Yaden, David B., Khoa D. Le Nguyen, Margaret L. Kern, Alexander B. Belser, Johannes C. Eichstaedt, Jonathan Iwry, et al. 2016. "Of Roots and Fruits: A Comparison of Psychedelic and Nonpsychedelic Mystical Experiences." *Journal of Humanistic Psychology* 57 (4): 338–353. doi:10.1177/0022167816674625.

28. Griffiths, R. R., W. A. Richards, U. McCann, and R. Jesse. 2006. "Psilocybin Can Occasion Mystical-Type Experiences Having Substantial and Sustained Personal Meaning and Spiritual Significance." *Psychopharmacology* 187 (3): 268–283. doi:10.1007/s00213-006-0457-5.

29. Muttoni, Silvia, Maddalena Ardissino, and Christopher John. 2019. "Classical Psychedelics for the Treatment of Depression and Anxiety: A Systematic Review." *Journal of Affective Disorders* 258: 11–24. doi:10.1016/j.jad.2019.07.076.

Chapter 16

1. Miller, Andrew C., Brandon K. Pfeffer, Michael R. Lawson, Kerry A. Sewell, Alexandra R. King, and Shahriar Zehtabchi. 2019. "Intravenous Magnesium Sulfate to Treat Acute Headaches in the Emergency Department: A Systematic Review." *Headache: Journal of Head and Face Pain* 59 (10): 1674–1686. doi:10.1111/head.13648.

2. Cevoli, Sabina, Valentina Favoni, and Pietro Cortelli. 2019. "Energy Metabolism Impairment in Migraine." *Current Medicinal Chemistry* 26 (34): 6253–6260. doi:10.2174/092986732566 6180622154411.

3. Gazerani, Parisa. 2020. "Migraine and Diet." *Nutrients* 12 (6): 1658. doi:10.3390/nu12061658; Razeghi Jahromi, Soodeh, Zeinab Ghorbani, Paolo Martelletti, Christian Lampl, and Mansoureh Togha. 2019. "Association of Diet and Headache." *Journal of Headache and Pain* 20 (1). doi:10.1186/s10194-019-1057-1.

4. Mitchell, Natasha, Catherine E. Hewitt, Shalmini Jayakody, Muhammad Islam, Joy Adamson, Ian Watt, and David J. Torgerson. 2011. "Randomised Controlled Trial of Food Elimination Diet Based on IgG Antibodies for the Prevention of Migraine Like Headaches." *Nutrition Journal* 10 (1). doi:10.1186/1475-2891-10-85; Hindiyeh, Nada Ahmad, Niushen Zhang, Mallory Farrar, Pixy Banerjee, Louise Lombard, and Sheena K. Aurora. 2020. "The Role of Diet and Nutrition in Migraine Triggers and Treatment: A Systematic Literature Review." *Headache: The Journal of Head and Face Pain* 60 (7): 1300–1316. doi:10.1111/head.13836.

5. Napadow, Vitaly. 2020. "The Mindful Migraine: Does Mindfulness-Based Stress Reduction Relieve Episodic Migraine?" *Pain* 161 (8): 1685–1687. doi:10.1097/j.pain.0000000000001859.

6. Barber, Mark, and Anna Pace. 2020. "Exercise and Migraine Prevention: A Review of the Literature." *Current Pain and Headache Reports* 24 (8). doi:10.1007/s11916-020-00868-6.

7. Lee, Hye Jeong, Jin Hyeok Lee, Eun Young Cho, Sun Mi Kim, and Seoyoung Yoon. 2019. "Efficacy of Psychological Treatment for Headache Disorder: A Systematic Review and Meta-Analysis." *Journal of Headache and Pain* 20 (1). doi:10.1186/s10194-019-0965-4; Nestoriuc, Yvonne, and Alexandra Martin. 2007. "Efficacy of Biofeedback for Migraine: A Meta-Analysis." *Pain* 128 (1): 111–127. doi:10.1016/j.pain.2006.09.007.

8. Chaibi, Aleksander, Peter J. Tuchin, and Michael Bjørn Russell. 2011. "Manual Therapies for Migraine: A Systematic Review." *Journal of Headache and Pain* 12 (2): 127–133. doi:10.1007/s10194-011-0296-6.

9. Flynn, Niamh. 2018. "Systematic Review of the Effectiveness of Hypnosis for the Management of Headache." *International Journal of Clinical and Experimental Hypnosis* 66 (4): 343–352. doi:10.1080/00207144.2018.1494432.

10. Urits, Ivan, Megha Patel, Mary Elizabeth Putz, Nikolas R. Monteferrante, Diep Nguyen, Daniel An, et al. 2020. "Acupuncture and Its Role in the Treatment of Migraine Headaches." *Neurology and Therapy* 9 (2): 375–394. doi:10.1007/s40120-020-00216-1.

11. Newberg, Andrew B., Patrick J. LaRiccia, Bruce Y. Lee, John T. Farrar, Lorna Lee, and Abass Alavi. 2005. "Cerebral Blood Flow Effects of Pain and Acupuncture: A Preliminary Single-Photon Emission Computed Tomography Imaging Study." *Journal of Neuroimaging* 15 (1): 43–49. doi:10.1111/j.1552-6569.2005.tb00284.x.

12. Puljak, Livia. 2019. "Can Botulinum Toxin Help Prevent Migraine in Adults?" *American Journal of Physical Medicine & Rehabilitation* 98 (3): 245–246. doi:10.1097/phm.0000000000001131.

13. Ebrahimi-Monfared, Mohsen, Mojtaba Sharafkhah, Ali Abdolrazaghnejad, Abolfazl Mohammadbeigi, and Fardin Faraji. 2017. "Use of Melatonin versus Valproic Acid in Prophylaxis of Migraine Patients: A Double-Blind Randomized Clinical Trial." *Restorative Neurology and Neuroscience* 35 (4): 385–393. doi:10.3233/rnn-160704; Gonçalves, Andre Leite, Adriana Martini Ferreira, Reinaldo Teixeira Ribeiro, Eliova Zukerman, José Cipolla-Neto, and Mario Fernando Prieto Peres. 2016. "Randomised Clinical Trial Comparing Melatonin 3 Mg, Amitriptyline 25 Mg and Placebo for Migraine Prevention." *Journal of Neurology, Neurosurgery & Psychiatry* 87 (10): 1127–1132. doi:10.1136/jnnp-2016-313458.

14. Diener, H. C., V. W. Rahlfs, and U. Danesch. 2004. "The First Placebo-Controlled Trial of a Special Butterbur Root Extract for the Prevention of Migraine: Reanalysis of Efficacy Criteria." *European Neurology* 51 (2): 89–97. doi:10.1159/000076535.

Chapter 17

1. Ayubcha, Cyrus, Mona-Elisabeth Revheim, Andrew Newberg, Mateen Moghbel, Chaitanya Rojulpote, Thomas J. Werner, and Abass Alavi. 2020. "A Critical Review of Radiotracers in the Positron Emission Tomography Imaging of Traumatic Brain Injury: FDG, Tau, and Amyloid Imaging in Mild Traumatic Brain Injury and Chronic Traumatic Encephalopathy." *European Journal of Nuclear Medicine and Molecular Imaging.* 48 (2): 623–641. doi:10.1007/s00259-020-04926-4.

2. Amen, Daniel G., Kristen Willeumier, Bennet Omalu, Andrew Newberg, Cauligi Raghavendra, and Cyrus A. Raji. 2016. "Perfusion Neuroimaging Abnormalities Alone Distinguish National Football League Players from a Healthy Population." *Journal of Alzheimer's Disease* 53 (1): 237–241. doi:10.3233/jad-160207.

3. Bédard, Michel, Melissa Felteau, Dwight Mazmanian, Karilyn Fedyk, Rupert Klein, Julie Richardson, et al. 2003. "Pilot Evaluation of a Mindfulness-Based Intervention to Improve Quality of Life among Individuals Who Sustained Traumatic Brain Injuries." *Disability and Rehabilitation* 25 (13): 722–731. doi:10.1080/0963828031000090489.

4. Leddy, John J., Mohammad N. Haider, Michael Ellis, and Barry S. Willer. 2018. "Exercise Is Medicine for Concussion. *Current Sports Medicine Reports* 17 (8): 262-270. doi:10.1249/jsr.0000000000000505.

5. O'Neil-Pirozzi, Therese M., and Henry Hsu. 2016. "Feasibility and Benefits of Computerized Cognitive Exercise to Adults with Chronic Moderate-to-Severe Cognitive Impairments following an Acquired Brain Injury: A Pilot Study." *Brain Injury* 30 (13–14): 1617–1625. doi:10.1080/02699052.2016.1199906.

6. Munivenkatappa, Ashok, Jamuna Rajeswaran, Bhagavatula Indira Devi, Niranjana Bennet, and Neeraj Upadhyay. 2014. "EEG Neurofeedback Therapy: Can It Attenuate Brain Changes in TBI?" *Neurorehabilitation* 35 (3): 481–484. doi:10.3233/nre-141140.

7. Stilling, Joan, Eric Paxman, Leah Mercier, Liu Shi Gan, Meng Wang, Farnaz Amoozegar, Sean P. Dukelow, Oury Monchi, and Chantel Debert. 2020. "Treatment of Persistent Post-Traumatic Headache and Post-Concussion Symptoms Using Repetitive Transcranial Magnetic Stimulation: A Pilot, Double-Blind, Randomized Controlled Trial." *Journal of Neurotrauma* 37 (2): 312–323. doi:10.1089/neu.2019.6692.

Chapter 18

1. Langa, Kenneth M., and Deborah A. Levine. 2014. "The Diagnosis and Management of Mild Cognitive Impairment." *JAMA* 312 (23): 2551. doi:10.1001/jama.2014.13806.

2. Tangalos, Eric G., and Ronald C. Petersen. 2018. "Mild Cognitive Impairment in Geriatrics." *Clinics in Geriatric Medicine* 34 (4): 563–589. doi:10.1016/j.cger.2018.06.005.

3. Rygiel, K. 2016. "Can Angiotensin-Converting Enzyme Inhibitors Impact Cognitive Decline in Early Stages of Alzheimer's Disease? An Overview of Research Evidence in the Elderly Patient Population." *Journal of Postgraduate Medicine* 62 (4): 242. doi:10.4103/0022-3859.188553.

4. Samant, Nikita Patil, and Girdhari Lal Gupta. 2020. "Novel Therapeutic Strategies for Alzheimer's Disease Targeting Brain Cholesterol Homeostasis." *European Journal of Neuroscience.* doi:10.1111/ejn.14949.

5. Amini, Yasmin, Nabeel Saif, Christine Greer, Hollie Hristov, and Richard Isaacson. 2020. "The Role of Nutrition in Individualized Alzheimer's Risk Reduction." *Current Nutrition Reports* 9 (2): 55–63. doi:10.1007/s13668-020-00311-7.

6. Farghali, Mahitab, Sara Ruga, Vera Morsanuto, and Francesca Uberti. 2020. "Can Brain Health Be Supported by Vitamin D-Based Supplements? A Critical Review." *Brain Sciences* 10 (9): 660. doi:10.3390/brainsci10090660.

7. Ramli, Nur Zuliani, Mohamad Fairuz Yahaya, Ikuo Tooyama, and Hanafi Ahmad Damanhuri. 2020. "A Mechanistic Evaluation of Antioxidant Nutraceuticals on Their Potential against Age-Associated Neurodegenerative Diseases." *Antioxidants* 9 (10): 1019. doi:10.3390/antiox9101019.

8. Browne, D., McGuinness, B., Woodside, J. V., and McKay, G. J. (2019). "Vitamin E and Alzheimer's Disease: What Do We Know So Far?" *Clinical Interventions in Aging*, 14, 1303–1317. https://doi.org/10.2147/CIA.S186760.

9. Wang, Rosy, and R. M. Damian Holsinger. 2018. "Exercise-Induced Brain-Derived Neurotrophic Factor Expression: Therapeutic Implications for Alzheimer's Dementia." *Ageing Research Reviews* 48: 109–121. doi:10.1016/j.arr.2018.10.002.

10. Troussière, Anne-Cécile, Christelle Monaca Charley, Julia Salleron, Florence Richard, Xavier Delbeuck, Philippe Derambure, et al. 2014. "Treatment of Sleep Apnoea Syndrome Decreases Cognitive Decline in Patients with Alzheimer's Disease." *Journal of Neurology, Neurosurgery & Psychiatry* 85 (12): 1405–1408. doi:10.1136/jnnp-2013-307544.

11. McClam, Tamela D., Christopher M. Marano, Paul B. Rosenberg, and Constantine G. Lyketsos. 2015. "Interventions for Neuropsychiatric Symptoms in Neurocognitive Impairment Due to Alzheimer's Disease." *Harvard Review of Psychiatry* 23 (5): 377–393. doi:10.1097/hrp.0000000000000097.

12. Luders, Eileen, Arthur W. Toga, Natasha Lepore, and Christian Gaser. 2009. "The Underlying Anatomical Correlates of Long-Term Meditation: Larger Hippocampal and Frontal Volumes of Gray Matter." *Neuroimage* 45 (3): 672–678. doi:10.1016/j.neuroimage.2008.12.061.

13. Eyre, Harris A., Bianca Acevedo, Hongyu Yang, Prabha Siddarth, Kathleen Van Dyk, Linda Ercoli, and Amber M. Leaver et al. 2016. "Changes in Neural Connectivity and Memory Following a Yoga Intervention for Older Adults: A Pilot Study." *Journal of Alzheimer's Disease* 52 (2): 673–684. doi:10.3233/jad-150653.

14. Khondoker, Mizanur, Snorri Bjorn Rafnsson, Stephen Morris, Martin Orrell, and Andrew Steptoe. 2017. „Positive and Negative Experiences of Social Support and Risk of Dementia in Later Life: An Investigation Using the English Longitudinal Study of Ageing." *Journal of Alzheimer's Disease* 58 (1): 99–108. doi:10.3233/jad-161160.

15. Lin, Kun-Pei, Yi-Chun Chou, Jen-Hau Chen, Chi-Dan Chen, Sheng-Ying Yang, Ta-Fu Chen, and Yu Sun et al. 2015. "Religious Affiliation and the Risk of Dementia in Taiwanese Elderly." *Archives of Gerontology and Geriatrics* 60 (3): 501–506. doi:10.1016/j.archger.2015.01.009; Khalsa, Dharma Singh. 2015. „Stress, Meditation, and Alzheimer's Disease Prevention: Where the Evidence Stands." *Journal of Alzheimer's Disease* 48 (1): 1–12. doi:10.3233/jad-142766.

16. Vakhapova, Veronika, Tzafra Cohen, Yael Richter, Yael Herzog, Yossi Kam, and Amos D. Korczyn. 2014. „Phosphatidylserine Containing Omega-3 Fatty Acids May Improve Memory Abilities in Nondemented Elderly Individuals with Memory Complaints: Results from an Open-Label Extension Study." *Dementia and Geriatric Cognitive Disorders* 38 (1–2): 39–45. doi:10.1159/000357793.

17. Monti, Daniel A., George Zabrecky, Thomas P. Leist, Nancy Wintering, Anthony J. Bazzan, Tingting Zhan, and Andrew B. Newberg. 2020. "N-Acetyl Cysteine Administration Is Associated with Increased Cerebral Glucose Metabolism in Patients with Multiple Sclerosis: An Exploratory Study." *Frontiers in Neurology* 11. doi:10.3389/fneur.2020.00088.

18. Witte, A. V., L. Kerti, D. S. Margulies, and A. Floel. 2014. "Effects of Resveratrol on Memory Performance, Hippocampal Functional Connectivity, and Glucose Metabolism in Healthy Older Adults." *Journal of Neuroscience* 34 (23): 7862–7870. doi:10.1523/jneurosci.0385-14.2014.

19. Bookheimer, Susan Y., Brian A. Renner, Arne Ekstrom, Zhaoping Li, Susanne M. Henning, Jesse A. Brown, et al. 2013. «Pomegranate Juice Augments Memory and FMRI Activity in Middle-Aged and Older Adults with Mild Memory Complaints." *Evidence-Based Complementary and Alternative Medicine* 2013: 1–14. doi:10.1155/2013/946298.

20. Lee, Juyoun, Byong Hee Choi, Eungseok Oh, Eun Hee Sohn, and Ae Young Lee. 2016. "Treatment of Alzheimer's Disease with Repetitive Transcranial Magnetic Stimulation Combined with Cognitive Training: A Prospective, Randomized, Double-Blind, Placebo-Controlled Study." *Journal of Clinical Neurology* 12 (1): 57. doi:10.3988/jcn.2016.12.1.57.

21. Im, Jooyeon Jamie, Hyeonseok Jeong, Marom Bikson, Adam J. Woods, Gozde Unal, Jin Kyoung Oh, and Seunghee Na et al. 2019. "Effects of 6-Month At-Home Transcranial Direct Current Stimulation on Cognition and Cerebral Glucose Metabolism in Alzheimer's Disease." *Brain Stimulation* 12 (5): 1222–1228. doi:10.1016/j.brs.2019.06.003.

22. Fotuhi, M., Lubinski, B., Trullinger, M., Hausterman, N., Riloff, T., Hadadi, M., & Raji, C. A. (2016). "A Personalized 12-Week 'Brain Fitness Program' for Improving Cognitive Function and Increasing the Volume of Hippocampus in Elderly with Mild Cognitive Impairment." *the Journal of Prevention of Alzheimer's Disease*, 3(3), 133–137. https://doi.org/10.14283/jpad.2016.92

23. Rosenberg, Anna, Alina Solomon, Tiia Ngandu, Esko Levälahti, Tiina Laatikainen, Teemu Paajanen, and Tuomo Hänninen et al. 2017. "Multidomain Lifestyle Intervention Benefits a Large Elderly Population at Risk for Cognitive Decline: Subgroup Analyses of the Finnish Geriatric Intervention Study to Prevent Cognitive Impairment and Disability (FINGER)." *Alzheimer's & Dementia* 13 (7): P239–P240. doi:10.1016/j.jalz.2017.06.086.

INDEX